The
Good Birth
Companion

To Ed – who gave me the little ones that started it all.

The
Good Birth
Companion

Your Essential Guide to Having
the Best Labour and Birth

Nicole Croft

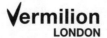

Vermilion
LONDON

1 3 5 7 9 10 8 6 4 2

Published in 2011 by Vermilion, an imprint of Ebury Publishing
A Random House Group company

The Random House Group Limited Reg. No. 954009

Addresses for companies within the Random House Group can be
found at www.randomhouse.co.uk

A CIP catalogue record for this book is available from the British Library

The Random House Group Limited supports The Forest Stewardship
Council (FSC), the leading international forest certification organisation.
All our titles that are printed on Greenpeace approved FSC certified
paper carry the FSC logo. Our paper procurement policy
can be found at www.randomhouse.co.uk

Mixed Sources
Product group from well-managed
forests and other controlled sources
www.fsc.org Cert no. TT-COC-2139
© 1996 Forest Stewardship Council

Printed in the UK by CPI Mackays, Chatham, ME5 8TD

ISBN 9780091935504

To buy books by your favourite authors and register for offers visit
www.randomhouse.co.uk

Inside illustrations: Stephen Dew

CONTENTS

FOREWORD

DR YEHUDI GORDON, FEBRUARY 2011

Since the 1980s active birth has been an important element of choice in the United Kingdom. Many hospitals and many midwives have taken on the active birth philosophy and have applied it to how they support women during labour and birth. However, the rapidly rising Caesarean section rate reflects changes in obstetric care and very importantly changes in consumer demand. This has resulted in a system with multiple rules during labour and birth and these may sometimes impede the active birth that many women seek.

This book will provide you with information and practical advice to help you navigate such a system, and find a way through the rules and regulations in the UK. It has been very well researched by Nicole, who has had experience both of giving birth herself and also of supporting and teaching many women to prepare for birth. The tone of the book is both warm and friendly and there are useful practical tips summarised at the end of each chapter.

Reading this book made me nostalgic for my involvement in the active birth movement since 1980. Medical understanding of the importance of a safe, warm and supportive environment has improved over time. We now know that a woman's intuition to give birth in a safe place helps the release of love hormones, natural painkillers and mothering hormones. This wonderful hormonal array is present in every woman and baby and when the circumstances are right the hormones flow in perfect symphony, with the mother/baby dyad at the centre. In the birth room everyone from the expectant father to the midwife is likewise bathed in these hormones. That is why an active and natural birth is so good for everyone involved.

This book is a very worthwhile addition to the choices available to women as they prepare for birth.

INTRODUCTION

'Don't be satisfied with stories, how things have gone with others. Unfold your own myth.'
Rumi

Every birth is different. There is no such thing as a blueprint for labour or a perfect birth, and there are as many different possible births as there are babies. There are, however, contrary to the story we are often told, many ways to significantly improve your birth experience and to greatly increase the chance that you will have a positive, even an empowering, experience. No birth is predestined. You can, and should, be in the driving seat.

It cannot be overemphasised, the extent to which a woman needs to prepare for birth. I confess I am still surprised at the number of women who don't so much as glance sideways at a book, and even more surprised when they go on to express shock that they found their labour difficult. Imagine embarking on a marathon without having given it a moment's thought? Or scaling a mountain without adequate physical and mental preparation?

...

We are very well equipped for labour. Nature is cleverly designed. Our hormones are finely tuned, our pelvises flexible and accommodating. The modern woman is usually in much better physical health than her forebears were, well nourished and healthy. We are also more educated, more inquiring and therefore potentially more informed. Coupled with this, medical advances have ensured that if things should go wrong, we have the back-up of a fantastic safety net: doctors and obstetricians who can perform emergency Caesareans and nurture premature babies, with staggering survival rates. In many ways, we should be counting our blessings, and the vast majority of women should be having incredibly positive birth experiences. Yet too many are not.

Too many of us are let down by a culture that sees birth as a medical condition and a system that has interfered with the process to such an extent that it no longer knows what birth really can be like. And it is a system that is truly overburdened. All around the country overworked and underpaid midwives are running between women in labour, unable to give them the emotional support that they know they need. All too often, monitoring is left to the machines. Epidurals are handed out for the good of the hospital, rather than the mother and baby, and the quality of a woman's birth has become simply a postcode lottery, entirely dependent on which of the very varied care happens to be on offer where she lives. And almost wherever you go, it seems, unnecessary intervention in the birth process is rife.

If all the interventions were necessary, if they made birth unequivocally safer, then the medicalisation of birth would not be a problem. It could simply be accepted as part of the evolutionary nature of things; out with the old, in with the new. We could look back on natural birth with nostalgia, but not with regret. But as we have learned from agriculture and the environment, we cannot meddle with nature without consequence. Countless scientific studies now testify to the fact that one intervention in the birth process tends to lead to another – the so-called 'cascade of intervention'. All too often, interventions are drafted in to solve a problem that they created in the first place.

For some women, an entirely impersonal, very medical birth experience imposed upon them makes no real difference. Some even actively court it, scheduling inductions and Caesareans to suit. But others, a huge number of others, feel entirely robbed of an experience they instinctively know should be more than just a procedure.

The very good news is that it doesn't have to be like this. The cult of questioning has begun. A generation ago women knew very little about birth; scans weren't available, antenatal classes were almost non-existent and, unless they had somehow managed to get hold of a copy of Grantly Dick-Read's *Childbirth Without Fear*, mothers went into labour on little more than a wing and a prayer, at best hyperventilating their way through the experience. Now, more and more women are less inclined to simply hand themselves over to the medical establishment without question. They want to have a part to play in their own experience. Empowerment, confidence, call it what you will – everywhere women are beginning to seek out information. It is, admittedly, not always easy. There is no doubt that where you happen to live

...

affects the choices available to you, and continuity of care may only be an option for those who can afford it. Water births are easily available in some places and more or less non-existent in others. Even the savviest mother might have to hunt high and low to find one. But I can assure you that if you understand how birth is meant to be, how it can and should be for the vast majority, you can make moves, however small, to create a better experience for yourself. For example, you might use the bed as a prop rather than a place to lie down; think carefully about who would be the best birth partner or find yourself a doula (see page 73); find a yoga for pregnancy class and get your breathing down to a fine art. What is truly amazing about birth is that the smallest things can make the biggest difference.

The truth is your body knows what to do. Ultimately, it will birth your baby, with or without you. What we need to do is start believing this. The Booker Prize-winning author Ben Okri once wrote that we are the stories we tell ourselves.[1] Our birth stories need to change.

We, individually and collectively, need to recognise the extraordinary capacity of women in their role as child bearers. We need to truly and properly understand the process of a natural birth. We need to recognise the importance of a woman's state of mind and that support is crucial to it. We need to understand a woman's body, its make-up and potential, the way in which labour unfolds and the cocktail of hormones that control it. We need to recognise that we are at once robust – women in comas have successfully given birth[2] – but that the process is also delicate; an unwanted visitor in the room, for example, can all but stop labour in its tracks. We need to recognise that our environment affects our mind, and that this in turn affects our body. And, finally, we need to recognise that good birth experiences are not simply down to luck; the choices we make have a material impact. Of course, there are no guarantees and there is no such thing as a perfect birth. One woman's idea of heaven is another's version of hell. Nature can always throw us a curve ball and, however well you prepare, you need also to arm yourself with an open mind and a willingness to change according to circumstances. But with the right information, good emotional support, an appropriate environment and a positive mindset, more women will secure themselves an experience that empowers them, and sets them off on the journey of motherhood very much on the front foot.

This book is intended to guide you through your birth preparation. It is, quite deliberately, not a trip through the nuts and bolts of a medicalised labour. I genuinely believe that birth, for the vast majority of women, is not a medical condition that needs to be fixed by a doctor. And if it becomes such, then knowing what a pair of forceps looks like in advance is not going to help you. When we go and have our appendix out, does an example of the scalpel help us get our heads round the idea? I suspect not. Whereas the previous generation of women suffered from not knowing enough about what was happening to their bodies during labour and birth, we now often suffer from knowing too much, and too much of the wrong things.

This book will fix that. It is a distillation of what I believe to be essential to the birth process and hope will make a huge difference to your understanding of labour and, crucially, of your role in it. It is based on almost 10 years of teaching real women from every walk of life, and with really positive results. Mothers very often come to me knowing very little and feeling utterly terrified. The vast majority leave with their heads held high, full of trust in their bodies and themselves.

The hope is that, like my classes, this book informs rather than bombards you, offering up information that will genuinely change your understanding of birth for the better. It is designed to empower you rather than frighten you. All too often our ideas about birth have been gleaned from ratings-driven TV dramas or the horror stories that women seem so keen to share. Rarely have any of us seen a birth first-hand. Rarely do we hear the amazing stories of the women who took back their experiences and made them their own, the ones who surprised themselves by their resilience and their strength, and their ability to birth with little or no intervention. And yet those women exist. They are all over the world, giving birth every single day. They also come back to my classes, on a very regular basis, and help to change the minds of the mothers who are still sitting, with their burgeoning bellies and it all ahead of them.

The book is split into three parts. The first part is the birth preparation, which will help you understand the birth process – not in terms of timelines and figures and protocols, but in terms of the physiology of birth, how the brain and the body work during labour and what this implies about the setting we should birth in. It will also give you what I believe is the key to any good birth preparation: an intimate understanding of the link between the body and the mind. This link is all too often undervalued in the modern maternity system, yet alive and well whenever we are dealing with anything that might be classified as instinctive behaviour. We will also talk about the normality and common sense of being active during labour and birth, the huge influence – both good and bad – of the people who support you and the benefits of using something as simple as water to facilitate the birth process. In essence, we will see how that much-used and thoroughly modern adage 'location, location, location' really applies to birth – but not necessarily in the way you might think.

The second part of the book deals with the birth itself. It is split into the three stages of labour, but the emphasis is still very much on the continuum that is any birth. The markers which I will give you are guides only, and nowhere is there an emphasis on commonly referred-to rules of thumb of the '1 cm, one hour' ilk, which all too often misguide even the most experienced midwife.

There is particular emphasis, as in the first section, on the things that I don't think anyone tells you, and yet which can fundamentally influence whether you might cope at a particular stage or not. Knowing what might happen and what is entirely normal is invaluable for when you are in labour itself.

By the end of the first and second part the book you should be able to write up a good birth plan. Not of the tick-box, downloaded template kind, that talks about whether you do or don't want to suck on gas and air at some point, but about the who's, the how's and the where's. This is all the big stuff. This is what matters. The other bits are – if I am completely honest – just window dressing.

And then the third part of the book is focused on the period just beyond the birth, from the hours that follow to those days and weeks and early months that women say they are often wholly underprepared for. All too often mothers complain that they were so focused on the birth that they forgot to think about what comes after it. And yet the birth is usually only half a day's experience. At the extreme, you might be labouring on and off for a few days but, in the whole scheme of things, it is not very long. So while preparation for such an almighty act is essential, it is also important to see the birth in context, as part of a much bigger journey that begins with conception and pregnancy and continues on into the all-consuming trip that is motherhood.

PART 1
Preparing for Birth

CHAPTER 1

The Monkey Puzzle
Birth and the Primal Brain

*'The list of our disastrous failures, from forest obliteration
and oceanic pollution to the raising of the extinction rate a
thousandfold, bears all the hallmarks of a species which no
longer believes itself to be a part of the animal world at all.
We're becoming unearthly, freed, we like to think, from the
physical imperatives of nature by technology and exiled from
its sensuality and immediacy by our own self-awareness.
Our role on the planet is compromised less by our power than
by this arrogance, and the belief that our particular brand of
consciousness makes us uniquely privileged as a species, entitled
to evaluate and manage the lives of all others on our own terms.'*
Richard Mabey, *Nature's Cure*

There is a very funny postcard that you might have come across,
featuring a line drawing of a heavily pregnant woman. She is
sweating and panting and clearly in the throes of labour, and in
the little speech bubble she proclaims, 'I've changed my mind'!
It's a funny little scene, primarily because we know that changing
her mind is not an option. When it comes to the eleventh hour,

.....

or the ninth month to be specific, the birth will happen, and it will happen with or without you. What we don't often think about, though, is how reassuring that is.

The truth is, after we have had a hand in the conception bit, everything else is down to nature. I have always found it remarkable that throughout an entire pregnancy we do very little and yet we grow an entire person. Of course there are aches and pains and unimaginable tiredness. Sometimes pregnancy feels like very hard work. And we can help the process along by staying healthy, avoiding certain foods and taking our folic acid but, for the most part, it is our bodies that create our babies.

A natural birth is just the same. It is the result of a concoction of hormones, working in their own time and their own way, which create the conditions that take a baby from the womb to the world. Believe it or not, a woman's body absolutely knows what to do. We don't need to think about it, or make it happen. It is important that we understand the process and that we create the conditions that are conducive to it, but also, crucially, that we don't get in the way.

It is rare that we think of ourselves as animals. We might subscribe to Darwin's theory of evolution, marvel at the idea of our 97 per cent shared genes with chimpanzees and even recognise animal behaviour in football hooligans, but the truth is most of us consider ourselves as separate from the animal kingdom. And there is no doubt that what sets us apart from animals is the cause for most of our celebrations. Our more sophisticated brain is what has given rise to our rich culture, our scientific breakthroughs, our inventiveness and our poetry. The world would be a decidedly blander, less colourful and much quieter place if it were not for our having developed an extraordinary number of extra brain cells. But for the purposes of birth, we need to think of ourselves as animals once more, for birth is about as primal as it gets.

Often we think of birth as a purely physical act, but it is essential that we also understand the mental side of birth. The birth you will have is not predestined. It is not stored deep in your DNA as a fait accompli, but can actually be wholly influenced – both positively and negatively – by your state of mind and your environment.

Birth and the Brain

In *very* rudimentary terms we can split the human brain into two parts. There is the primal brain, made up of the hindbrain and the limbic system, and this is the part of the brain that we share with other mammals. This is our animal brain. The second part is the front brain, the neo-cortex, which we share with higher-level animals, but which is decidedly bigger in humans. In fact, this part makes up to two-thirds of the human brain. We mainly live in this latterly developed part of the brain – this is where we think, deduce, plan, rationalise and problem-solve. It is our neo-cortex that enables us to solve complex mathematical equations, compose symphonies, design buildings and even write a shopping list. By comparison, the instinctive brain lies fairly dormant, quietly taking care of our reflexes and most of our social taboos: sexual activity, bowel movements, hunger and thirst. While the primal brain tends to take a back seat most of the time in modern life, it needs to come into its own for the purposes of birth.

When an unborn baby's lungs are fully developed, a hormonal signal is sent to the mother's primal brain, which in turn emits a cocktail of hormones, including oxytocin and prostaglandins, to instigate labour. These hormones, which change in combination and composition throughout the whole of the birth, are responsible for everything that follows. They are intricate, delicately balanced and worthy of awe. They can also, however, be interrupted by medical intervention or – and this is the key – by the 'switching on' of the front brain in any way. For though the different parts of the brain exist side by side, they struggle to function in tandem.

To give you an example: imagine you are staying in a remote cottage in the Highlands of Scotland. You wake up in the middle of the night needing the toilet. Bleary-eyed, you get out of bed and stumble out towards the bathroom. As you do, you tread on something unexpected. Alarmed, you pull your foot back and look down. Something long and thin is stretched across the doorway – a snake! Your heart begins to beat faster, your mouth goes dry, your pupils dilate and you have a sudden urge to run. Your perception of danger has sparked a physiological response that comes directly from the primal brain. A huge surge of adrenaline has been produced and your body is responding accordingly. The fact that snakes are rare in the Highlands and that you haven't even seen it properly is irrelevant at the moment your instincts kick in. Your intellect has been momentarily repressed. Your primal brain is working without recourse to your rationality.

Your scream wakes up your friend who runs out of his room and turns on the light. You – still white faced, with pulse racing – look down to see that by your foot is an old piece of rope. Your heartbeat begins to slow, blood returns to your face and you grimace with mild embarrassment. Reason is restored, and there is no need to be afraid.

So, instincts can override reason – if you need further proof, think back to your behaviour as a loved-up teenager! But in the same way that instincts can induce irrationality, reason can also smother instinct. And as evolution has accorded us a more sophisticated brain, it seems that our instincts have been increasingly marginalised. In fact, when it comes to birth the rational brain is the veritable playground bully, dominating and impeding the functioning of the primal, instinctive brain to detrimental effect.

So if the two parts of the brain can't work in tandem, and the front or thinking brain is the bully, we need to think about birth in terms of actually switching off that front brain and allowing the back brain, our instinctive animal brain, to work on its own and unimpeded. How do we do this? How do we function, temporarily, in a more mammalian state?

The first step is to understand the physiology of birth and trust that our bodies will function as they ought to. With so much interference, it is difficult to distinguish between what is an inherent part of the birth process and what has been manipulated beyond recognition. A huge proportion of doctors and midwives now attend to births having never seen an unmanaged labour. In the Philippines, it is mandatory that obstetricians attend a certain number of home births as part of their training. In the UK, they have no such obligation. Many doctors who are against home births will admit, if pressed, that they have never been to one. The result is that instead of seeing birth as normal and natural, they regard it as a medical condition, one that needs to be monitored, supported and manipulated. If those who care for us have this view of birth, how are we – as mothers who come to birth with no prior experience of it – to know otherwise?

It is an essential part of the process of birth preparation that we seek to challenge this idea. If we accept that *birth is something that womankind has been doing successfully for generations*, that the female body is not misdesigned and that the vast majority of births can and should be positive experiences, we improve our chances that they will be. Most mothers, especially in the West, are healthy and have every reason to anticipate an uncomplicated birth. And the World Health Organization (WHO) suggests that the vast majority of births – up to 90 per cent – should be normal and uncomplicated.[3] That should be a more widely touted statistic. The problem is that representations of birth on TV and the inclination in our culture for emphasising the horror stories imply the opposite. During my last pregnancy, an arguably draconian doctor asked me if I would like to hear of a local horror story, by way of emphasising a particular danger. I politely but firmly declined. Faced with a similar antagonist you should do the same. Horror stories eat away at our capacity to trust ourselves, and if we can't trust, we can't let go. So go to a class where the emphasis is on positive birth stories. Find birth videos – your midwife should be able to recommend them – where you can see for yourself what a positive labour looks like. And when you watch them, do so twice. The first time you might be surprised at a real birth – it might well be noisier, messier and more primal than you first imagined. But on second viewing you will have absorbed everything, and chances are you will already see birth in a different way and be more comfortable with it.

Lastly, remember that for you to be here today it has taken generation after generation of mothers who have birthed their babies. Your baby knows what to do, and your body knows what to do.

The Natural Shutdown

Once we have recognised that birth is a process that women are actually quite good at, and certainly more than capable of, we need to try to shut down that front part of the brain – the chattering, thinking, planning, worrying part of the brain – to allow space for the back part to take the lead.

There is no doubt that this is easier said than done. The mind, as the Tibetans would say, can be an unruly monkey. As anyone who has tried to meditate will testify, 'switching off' is much easier in theory than it is in practice. We might well want to calm our mind and subdue our rationality, but usually our intellect will use any excuse – even a shopping list or plans for the weekend – to take over.

Rest assured, though: nature is on a mother's side on this one. It has long been a source of both amusement and frustration that pregnant women become more forgetful as their pregnancy progresses. In an Australian study, 82 per cent of the pregnant mothers surveyed reported some sort of absent-mindedness or inability to concentrate.[4] This, believe it or not, is a good thing. This 'pregnancy amnesia', as it is often referred to, is the result of hormonal changes that occur in preparation for labour. A small study has even claimed to show that the front brain decreases in size and the back brain, or more specifically the pituitary gland which is a part of it, actually increases by the same amount, all in preparation for it to take the lead during birth and early motherhood.[5] So the next time you put the keys in the fridge and find yourself walking to the car with a pound of butter, celebrate your forgetfulness as a good sign. It means that your mind is preparing for birth and is further proof that you are well designed for it.

Practice Makes Perfect

We can help this natural shutdown by using our pregnancy to practise switching off. That is why yoga for pregnancy classes are such a fantastic way to prepare for birth, as yoga works both on the body and, in particular, the mind, helping you to focus inwards, to be attentive to your breath, and to gradually still your thoughts. With regular practice, the act of switching off will come to you more and more easily. If you have access to a regular yoga for pregnancy class, then I highly recommend going to it – the midwives who work near me claim that they can tell if a woman has been practising yoga during pregnancy as she tends to be calmer and more centred throughout labour, and is capable of breathing her way rather beautifully through even the strongest of her contractions. If a class is not an option for you, then there are plenty of good yoga for pregnancy DVDs out there, which enable you to practise in your own time. As with all physical activity during pregnancy, make sure you okay it with your midwife before embarking on anything that is wholly new.

Hypnobirthing or natal hypnotherapy is another wonderful way to prepare for birth, for the same reason that it works on settling the mind, alleviating lurking fears and sowing positive mental seeds in their place. Fears and worries will keep the brain unnecessarily switched on and so will act as an impediment to an easy labour. Remove the fears, and your back brain is free to function.

Meditation is another good calming option and a fantastic way to subdue fears. It is rare to find classes that are designed specifically for pregnant women, but an ordinary class, or even a meditation CD, will help train the mind in the act of switching off.

Whatever method you choose, remember that switching off is a natural part of the birth process, so just allow it to happen. Many a mother who has known nothing about the theory will speak of 'feeling away with the fairies' during the birth, or of the 'timeless' quality of labour. Losing the ability to converse and to think rationally are part and parcel of a positive birth experience and a good sign that the intellectual brain is taking a back seat, as it should.

The Birth Environment

This natural shutting-down process can be helped along on the day with careful consideration of the environment you choose to birth in. The back brain functions better in certain environments, and less well in others. When it comes to designing your birth place, simply consider what conditions you need in order to sleep well. Because the best place to sleep is also the best place to labour. So what do you need to go to sleep best?

PRIVACY

First and foremost, you need privacy to give birth. It's nigh on impossible to sleep when you have an audience, and even harder to birth with one. Animals have this one all figured out. Herd animals, such as sheep or the rhesus monkey, naturally leave their group to give birth, coming back to join the crowd when they are done and dusted with their baby in tow. Anyone whose cat has given birth will know that when the time comes a cat will find somewhere private and enclosed to birth its kittens. And this mammalian need to feel unobserved for birth is universal. Stories abound of tribal cultures where women actually go to birth completely on their own. In many places, the culture is for women to have a small, designated hut that is considered the birthplace. These are often out of the way and are almost always all-female territories, where women feel the right balance of privacy and security to completely let themselves go and give themselves up to the birth process. And, again, this is instinct working at its best – Michel Odent, pioneering French obstetrician turned midwife, has often said that he absolutely knew a home birth was going well if he arrived to find an unsuspecting husband panic-stricken because his wife had locked herself in the bathroom and was refusing anyone entry. Endless are the stories of women who have given birth crammed into a toilet, because they say 'It's where I felt like being'. A small, dark and private place makes the perfect birth nest.

A woman in one of my classes had exactly this instinct. She had decided upon a hospital birth but intended to labour as much as she could at home. In preparation, she'd put beanbags, a birth ball and low-level lighting in her living room. She'd hoped – she later told me – to spend all her early labour in the room, with only her husband for support. But when it all kicked off, the specified birth nest lay empty. Instead, she found herself drawn upstairs to what she called her 'ironing room', which was effectively nothing more than an oversized cupboard, where she laboured happily for several hours until her husband insisted, eventually quite firmly, that they go to hospital. When they got there, after only five hours labouring across the ironing board, she was 8 cms dilated and only an hour and a half away from the birth of her first baby! Her instinct to find somewhere quiet and contained had clearly paid off.

By contrast, when I was working on the introduction to my yoga for pregnancy DVD and had to search through photographic archives day after day, I was horrified by the number of pictures of women lying, legs dramatically spread, spotlight poised, being peered at by half a dozen faces. In the face of this gawking, this hefty audience, is it at all surprising that the Western world is alone in speaking of births that last 36 hours and of women's bodies seemingly shutting down? (On that note, it is useful to think of the need for the mind to shut down, so that the body opens up – not the other way around.)

How easy is it to go to sleep with an audience? How can we assume that giving birth – a primal and intimate act – will be any more successful with an entourage? If men talk liberally of stage fright in urinals, shouldn't we consider the possibility of similar stage fright in delivery rooms? Ina May Gaskin, a celebrated American midwife, calls this the 'sphincter law'.[6] It sounds a rather base way of putting it, but her argument is that the laws at work during labour and birth are the same as those for excretion. If we need privacy for something as commonplace as a toilet stop, how can we assume that it is not equally necessary for the enormous, but also fundamental, act of birth? In all but an emergency situation, a woman should be entitled to give birth without an audience of strangers.

It has not been completely lost on the medical profession that strangers can be an impediment to birth. It's just that you have to

---

WHAT TO BRING TO A HOSPITAL BIRTH FOR A BETTER BIRTH ENVIRONMENT

- A sheet to hang at the window.
- A small lamp.
- A pillow and/or your own blanket.
- Birth music CDs or a well-stocked iPod (you might also need to bring the dock).
- Aromatherapy oils.
- Earplugs and/or eye mask.
- A birth ball.

delve as far back as the 1800s to find written evidence of it. Whereas modern textbooks are mute on the subject, the diaries of 19th-century physicians are enlightening. Many of them have records of times when their arrival at the home of a labouring woman coincided exactly with her labour stalling and, although it was often interrupted for several hours, in one rare instance the poor woman's labour stopped for a fortnight before starting again![7]

In fact, any look at births across cultures shows a strong positive correlation between how isolated a woman is to give birth and the ease of her delivery. And the converse is true, too – the more people a woman has to contend with, the longer the whole process seems to take. Birth is not, by any means, a team sport.

WHERE TO GIVE BIRTH

This fundamental need for security and privacy should inform your decision about where to give birth. The endless debates about whether the home or hospital is best assume that every woman needs the same environment. I genuinely believe that the black or white argument about home vs hospital misses the point. Where you give birth should be entirely dependent on where you, as an individual, will feel the safest. Not where your husband or mother or friend feels the safest, but where you do. For some mothers that will be where they know that medical intervention is on tap and an epidural only a corridor away. I have one good friend who positively relishes the opportunity to go to hospital for the births of her babies. She now has three children and on every occasion she had her bag packed well in advance and counted the days like a child before Christmas, so eager was she to be in a hospital bed and attended to by an entourage of kindly nurses. Other people – myself included – can't stand hospitals, associating them with the sick, and tense up the minute they step through the revolving doors. And tensing up is the exact opposite of what you want to be doing when you give birth. So make the decision that is right for you.

Do not simply assume that because the vast majority of women give birth in hospitals this makes them better for everyone. Huge studies have shown that for mothers with no previously flagged complications, birth at home is at least as safe as in a hospital. In fact, the largest recent study on home birth, published in 1997, showed that birthing at home halves your chances of having a Caesarean or forceps delivery.[8] Holland has a 30 per cent home birth rate and very low rates of maternal mortality – lower than the UK in fact.[9] Marsden Wagner, former head of the World Health Organization, goes as far as to say, 'If you really want a humanised birth, you need to get the hell out of the hospital.'[10] And the truth is, birth without intervention is far more likely at home. But, equally, don't opt for a home birth just because your friend is having one. Think it through and decide what is best for you. Where will *you* feel most safe and most secure? Because the answer to that question is the right place for you. If you do want a home birth, discuss it with your midwife. You are legally entitled to choose a home birth, but may encounter some resistance to the idea. If you are sure a home birth is what you want but don't seem to be making headway, ask to speak to the local supervisor of midwives or the midwife manager. Alternatively, contact AIMS (Association for Improvements in Maternity Services) (see page

268), who will be happy to give you information (they have a good leaflet entitled *Choosing a Home Birth*).

A happy medium for some women are birthing centres within hospitals, which have been shown to have less intervention than hospital births. They are usually less medical settings, staffed by midwives who are comfortable with natural births and with the security of conventional hospital care only a floor or building away. Women tend to speak in glowing terms about their experiences of birth centres. Your midwife will be a good first port of call if you want to find one. Ask her what your options are in the area. Antenatal and yoga for pregnancy teachers also usually know what is available, and many have a list of not just birth centres but also independent midwives and doulas. If you find a birth centre near you, then do your homework. Some are more autonomous than others and it is worth asking for a copy of their policy notes and comparing them to the hospitals to see if they are truly independent. In fact, it is advisable to ask for a copy of a hospital's policy notes wherever you plan to go. All too often, women have an idea of how they would like their birth to be, only to find their plans derailed by proclaimed protocols and arbitrary time limits. In the thick of labour, and unarmed with any prior knowledge, it is easy to be railroaded into saying yes to anything that is offered, regardless of whether you like it or not. Seeing the hospital notes in advance not only means you can manage your own expectations, but enables you to query things, if necessary, once you are on their territory. Another good source of information is the website BirthChoice UK (www.birth choiceuk.com), which provides hospital and birthing centre statistics. A good thing to look up is their intervention rates, but remember that the larger hospitals necessarily have more intervention as they care for both high-risk and low-risk mothers. Regardless, it will still give you a flavour of how the hospital operates and what its birth outcomes are.

DARKNESS

As well as feeling unobserved and secure, women tend to labour better when they are somewhere dimly lit. Darkness helps the process of shutting down, whereas light very specifically stimulates our front brain (see page 13). It is why, unless you are exhausted, it is nigh on impossible to get to sleep with the lights on. And, unsurprisingly, giving birth in the dark is a fairly common phenomenon. Animals largely give birth at night, as any bleary-eyed farmer will confirm during lambing in the spring. It is also very common for mothers to speak of a long early labour, that might well have started and stopped throughout the whole day, only to become truly established as the sun set. My sister-in-law had exactly that experience – she laboured on and off all day and got so bored that by the early evening she went with her partner to the pub for a change of scenery, at which point things really began to kick off. Luckily for the landlord, they decided on a speedy trip home rather than another round!

Midwives will tell you that they are at their busiest in the evening and early hours of the morning. The dark, it seems, is the natural environment for labour. And common sense suggests it could not be otherwise – think of the proverbial rabbit caught in the headlights (absolutely what we do not want to be while giving birth). Whenever we want to create a sense of privacy and atmosphere – be it an atmospheric dinner party or a romantic night in – we usually opt to turn down the lights. The darkness is where people generally, and labouring mothers especially, feel most protected, most at ease with nakedness and most unobserved.

If you are birthing at home, then your lighting choices are at your discretion. In hospital, creating low-level lighting can sometimes be more tricky, but it is by no means impossible. When you tour the hospital in late pregnancy, find out what provisions are made for lighting, and if there is nothing more on offer than a strip light, pack a small lamp in your hospital bag – stranger things have been taken in! Another option, which I used recently at a birth as a doula, was to turn the main lights off and open the door to allow in shafts of corridor light. This, coupled with the light from the birthing pool, was ample for the midwife to work and to write her notes, but dark enough that the mother felt enclosed and private. If you are in labour during the day, then it might be a good idea to put a sheet up at the window – it won't necessarily give you darkness, but it will subdue the light. Several women in my class also said they used an eye mask – the ones you get given on aeroplanes – but if you haven't packed one, or don't fancy being constricted, then simply closing your eyes can help you to retreat. So in whatever way you can, minimise bright lights, as they will make relaxing and switching off more difficult.

FAMILIARITY

We tend to be most comfortable and relaxed in familiar environments. When we are seeing something for the first time, our senses are switched on to high alert, taking in the novelty of the sights and sounds and smells in acute detail. Wherever you decide to give birth, make sure it is at least a little bit familiar. Visit at least once, though more if you can, because each visit will make you feel more at home. Most hospitals provide hospital tours, and some places will allow you to book your 36-week appointment there. If you have a choice, ask for your scans to be in the hospital you think you'd like to give birth in. I also advise women who are going to hospital to take things from home with them – a pillow that has the scent of their own washing powder or that very particular smell that you associate with home, as well as their own clothes and towels. In this way, your sense of smell can effectively switch off, numbed by the fact that it is engulfed by something it knows.

MINIMAL DISTURBANCE

If you are going to sleep, you want as little noise and talking as possible. A very common feature of a birth that moves from home is that on arrival at the hospital, labour tends to slow down for a time. Though bumpy car journeys and ill-timed traffic jams are often enough to stall even the most established labour, another culprit is likely to be the questions and form-filling that is required of the labouring mother when she arrives. The minute you are questioned, you are forced to switch on your thinking brain in order to answer. If you were near sleep, you'd have to wake up.

Immediately this will interrupt any rhythm you have had, and will, in all likelihood, slow or stall your labour for a time at least.

The best way around this is to assign the job of chief talker to your birth partner. You can then try to ignore your surroundings as much as possible by directing your senses inward and focusing on your breath. Look down, if necessary, leaning against a wall or over a chair. And when you are taken to where you will be labouring for a time, get back into whatever rhythm you found while at home, trying as much as possible to ignore everything around you. If music is going to block out unfamiliar sounds, then by all means plan to use it – just make sure your birth CD is long or you have a seemingly endless choice on your iPod, otherwise the fact that Neil Young's 'Harvest Moon' is playing for the 14th time might be enough to drive you insane. And, if not you, then certainly your birth partner! Equally, don't be surprised if sometimes you feel you'd prefer silence. If that is what you are after, then a set of earplugs might just do the trick, especially if you are labouring on an exceptionally busy ward. It's your labour you want to focus on, not anyone else's.

Another potential disturbance is any intervention in the birth process. Being advised, rigged up, turned over and generally poked and prodded is going to bring you out of your lovely labour stupor and have you thinking nineteen to the dozen. When intervention is truly necessary then quite frankly who cares which part of the brain you are inhabiting, but in all other circumstances, accept intervention cautiously. Again, have your partner question the relevance of anything you are offered so you can continue to focus inwards.

Internal examinations may not be unnecessary interventions, but they are bound to disturb you in some way. A vaginal examination (VE) is a procedure done by your midwife to measure your dilation. She will usually ask you to lie down and then put her hand, or several fingers, inside your vagina to feel the cervix. There are obvious benefits to the procedure – for the midwife it is sometimes good to measure your progress and, particularly at the end of the first stage, to make sure you are fully dilated. You might also want to know how you are progressing. But, remember, it is a disturbance of sorts, and you may not always get the answer you were hoping for. With this in mind, try to limit the number of examinations and ask the midwife to examine you upright or on all fours to avoid having to lie on your back. If the midwife insists you are semi-reclining, then rest assured the procedure is quick, and try to simply breathe deeply and relax. As soon as she is finished, return to your chosen position.

WARMTH

Feeling warm is less about the brain and more about the body, but is important nonetheless. It is essential that you are warm enough during labour. Just as it is difficult to go to sleep when it is cold, letting go is more difficult when you are struggling with the temperature. In the face of cooler temperatures the body tends to tense up, the shoulders lift and the chest draws in. As birth is all about opening up and letting go, being warm is essential. A pair of nice, warm socks can work wonders at regulating your body temperature, so add them to your hospital bag and ask for them if you are feeling nippy. Make sure you speak up if you are feeling too cold – or, indeed, too hot. Windows can easily be opened and shut, no matter what the time of year. And make sure that whatever your temperature you stay well hydrated, taking little sips of water or diluted cordial through a bendy straw.

At home, controlling your environment is easy, so the optimal conditions for birth – the privacy, the darkness, the familiarity and the warmth – can be created with ease. In a hospital setting these conditions are often desperately lacking and it is often up to you to make them happen. Though sitcoms misrepresent birth to an alarming degree, what they often get right is the bright lights, the mass of people, the stirrups and the machines. But it doesn't have to be like this.

Stipulate in your birth plan (see page 54) that you would like to create the best possible conditions for labour. Insist, if necessary, on having certain conditions in the room, and if you encounter resistance find out why. If the response is unconvincing, then ask your partner to request any changes you would like. Feel free to question who needs to be in the room. It is not uncommon for experienced midwives to banish doctors from the room of their own accord, unless their presence is truly necessary. But if your midwife is a little less forthright than you would like, again get your partner to question the presence of any additional people. In my regular workshops for couples, I suggest that the perfect role for partners – who often claim to feel like something of a spare part in hospital births – is to act as a buffer between you and the system. By being your voice, they can minimise your need to talk, allow you to retreat and leave you to just make only the sounds that you feel compelled to make instinctively. And, incidentally, no one should discourage your noises. They are both a natural and a necessary part of labour – and they can even be liberating. As one beautiful Spanish woman in my class once said, 'Birth is the only time you can get down on all fours, moo like a cow and be congratulated for it.' Some couples find it useful to have a 'code' between them – a nod or a wink or a word – which is the partner's cue to take charge or be assertive. If you think that would help, come up with something in advance – but make sure it is something your partner will definitely notice. The last thing you want to do is to be squinting frantically and frustratedly in the corner while your partner is smiling at you from afar!

The importance of a woman's state of mind and her surroundings is seeping, albeit slowly, into mainstream birth culture. Some women are lucky enough to have access to birthing centres or midwife-led units that have redesigned their delivery rooms to take into account a woman's primal needs. The people who run these centres usually have a fundamental understanding of the birth process, so their practices accord with their interior design choices. Many women find, however, that they need to battle to turn down the lights and get rid of the audience, even in apparently progressive hospitals. But as soon as we understand the process of birth, and the need to liberate the primal brain from the rein of the rational, we understand why the environment we birth in is more than just a matter of decoration.

SUMMARY

- We tend to think of birth as a purely bodily function, yet the mind also plays an essential role.
- Birth is controlled and directed by a cocktail of hormones that come from your back or 'animal' brain. To allow this to happen smoothly, you need to switch off your front brain.
- This dominance of the back brain happens to a degree on its own, hence the pregnancy amnesia you're bound to experience.
- The environment you birth in plays a huge part – the perfect place to give birth is also the perfect place to sleep.
- Decide where to give birth based on where *you* will feel the most secure.
- Make sure you are as familiar as you can be with your chosen place of birth, and bring items from home to enhance your sense of security.
- When the time comes, allow yourself to let go and retreat. Remember, meditators take years of practice to get into that part of the brain – you've got limited access to a fast track!

CHAPTER 2

Stand Up for Active Birth
Being Mobile in Labour

*'The day when Janet Balaskas introduced the phrase
"active birth" was possibly the most important one in
the history of childbirth in Europe.'*
Michel Odent

While birth is entirely instinctive, it is not in any way passive. Our mental images of birth, those that we have gleaned from books or from film scenes, suggest that we need to lie back and be delivered, but this could not be further from the truth. As medicine has gradually encroached upon birth, women have been increasingly both immobilised and sidelined, but the key to a positive birth is to get up and to put yourself back in the centre of your own experience. Being active, both physically and mentally, is essential to a good birth experience.

We live in a society that is undoubtedly obsessed with fashion and fad. One celebrity is seen in a particular pair of boots and suddenly the streets are awash with them. A season later, the clothes hanger of the day says they are no longer stylish and we willingly obey and banish the boots to the back of the closet. One person has the latest gadget, and then suddenly millions do. Last season it was the iPhone, now everyone is clamouring after the iPad. Though it would be reasonable to assume that something as important as birth would be immune to such flippant fad following, it is not. You only need look to Brazil, where it has become fashionable to have a Caesarean, to see the impact of trends on something as fundamental as birth. In some parts of urban Brazil, Caesarean rates are as high as 80 per cent.

Though the copycat culture has reached epic proportions in the 21st century, people have always been guided by the trends of the day. The act of lying down to give birth was said to have been one such trend. The myth is that, in pursuit of a better view of his illegitimate child's birth, Louis the 14th ordered his mistress to lie down to give birth. It then supposedly became a mark of great sophistication to lie down in a 'ladylike' fashion to give birth.

This may be nothing more than hearsay. It is perhaps more likely that lying down to give birth coincided with increasing intervention in the birth process and landmarks like the invention of forceps. As technology encroached upon birth and labours were increasingly medically managed, having women immobilised made it easier to control them. It is also possible that as male physicians took over, they were less inclined to adopt all manner of postures to accommodate an upright woman. Whatever the true origins of lying down to give birth, there is no doubt that the spread of this very irrational position was in part due to following a trend.

Active Birth Around the World

Since the beginning of time, women who have been left to labour instinctively have done so in a variety of upright and mobile positions. Left to her own devices, a woman will choose to squat, kneel, walk and sway her way through the first stage of labour. She will tend to roll her pelvis as though in a dance in an attempt to alleviate discomfort. Instinctively, she will circle her hips, mimicking and thus aiding the spiralling descent of the baby through the birth canal. Stories are often told of babies who seem to be stuck; the mother, intuitively feeling this, suddenly has a desire to walk up stairs or lift one leg, only to find she has 'miraculously' dislodged her baby who then arrives with considerable speed. One young woman, who coped admirably with a drawn-out labour at home, said that the only time she felt pain that was unmanageable was when she was encouraged to lie down, momentarily, to have an internal examination. 'I couldn't bear being on my back,' she said. 'As soon as the midwife was done I got up and refused to lie back again.'

Another woman in one of my classes, so petite that she looked as though a breath of wind might blow her over, recounted her birth story: 'I simply couldn't stay still. My labour seemed to develop its own rhythm and so did I. It was almost as if the birth was the music and I felt compelled to dance to it.' She managed, despite her slight frame, to 'dance' a very robust 9 lb 11 oz boy into the world, with no assistance at all.

History shows that this instinct to move, to be active in labour, is by no means new. Artistic representations of birth across cultures and throughout the ages depict women labouring and giving birth in upright positions. When an eccentric Englishman by the name of George Engelmann did an extensive global study of birth as far back as 1882, he came to the conclusion that lying down to give birth was a Western anomaly and suggested the reason for it could only be prudery. Highly politically incorrect, he refers to tribal people as savages. His book, *Labor Amongst Primitive People*,[11] is nevertheless considered a classic. As the only record of cross-cultural birth of the time, it is a unique and valuable insight into old birth practice. In it he shows that, contrary to popular belief, lying down was not the most common position that women adopted during labour. Though there was not a single birth position that dominated, upright squatting, all fours and kneeling tended to be the most commonly used whereas lying down was rarely, if ever.

A trawl through photographic archives shows that things have changed since Engelmann's day. The West has been very successful at exporting the rather unglamorous 'stranded beetle' position for labour (lying on your back with legs splayed). In places where birth has escaped overt management, women still give birth as they might have done generations ago, but wherever birth is more medicalised women now tend to lie down – sometimes on thin camp beds and in little rows, divided by little more than a thin curtain. In fact lying down for birth is so common that in many places, including parts of the UK, it's considered entirely normal or even appropriate.

In the 1970s, a pioneer by the name of Janet Balaskas began her own little revolution against lying down to give birth. Unnerved by what she saw as already unnecessary levels of birth intervention, she conducted a study of her own and discovered –

as Mr Engelmann had done almost 100 years earlier – that wherever birth was not managed, women laboured in a host of upright positions. Balaskas then went on to explore the physiology of the female pelvis and discovered that it was significantly compromised if a woman lay down. This led to her coining the phrase 'active birth' and to opening the now famous Active Birth Centre in North London (see page 268) from where she has set about re-educating hundreds of women about the benefits of being active in labour. And science has now caught up with her, showing that active births are shorter, less painful, less likely to need intervention and ultimately dramatically improve a woman's experience of birth.[12]

Why is an Active Birth Better?

1) MORE SPACE IN THE PELVIS

Anatomical studies have shown that there is up to 30 per cent more space in the pelvis when a woman is upright.[13] That is almost a third of the possible space, so huge! If there was no other reason to get up off your back, that would be reason alone.

During pregnancy a hormone called relaxin is produced, which softens the ligaments that hold the pelvis together, enabling it to expand during birth. In fact, you'd be surprised and heartened by how much extra space is gained and how mobile and open the pelvis actually is (and remember, too, that a baby's head is made of soft bones that can mould and move for birth). So it is not the case that a fixed object is moving through a fixed space – it is an altogether more malleable process.

A lot of the extra space in the pelvis comes from the flexibility of the coccyx, which is the little bony bit at the base of the spine – this is quite bendy and is capable of actually moving back and out of the way. When you're upright, this movement is possible and significantly increases the available space in your pelvic outlet to accommodate the head of the descending baby. In fact, so crucial is this extra space that in Jamaica midwives say 'a woman will only give birth when her back opens up'. If, however, you are labouring on your back, this opening of the sacrum is blocked and so all the potential extra space is lost.[14]

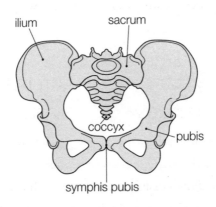

FEMALE PELVIS

The truth is, babies are designed to get through pelvises and it is rare, especially nowadays when nutrition is so improved and women's pelvises properly formed, that there isn't enough room. But it is still a tight fit, so you want to be sure that you are using every available bit of space. Being upright ensures you maximise the space in your pelvis and create an altogether easier journey for your baby.

2) HARNESSING THE BENEFITS OF GRAVITY

By being up on your knees or feet, gravity gives you a helping hand. You don't need to understand the details of Newton's physics to know that it is easier to push something down rather than push it up. It is simple common sense that to get a baby to descend through the birth canal is going to require less effort if you work with gravity rather than against it. In fact, an engineer father who came to one of my classes once did a nifty calculation that concluded giving birth to an average-sized baby while lying down was the physical equivalent to pushing out about 22 lb of weight. Youch! Get up, and you go back to birthing a baby whose average weight will be about 7½ lb.

3) BABY'S HEAD APPLIES PRESSURE ON THE CERVIX

Being upright enables the baby's head to apply even pressure on your cervix. This even and constant contact between head and cervix sends strong and consistent messages to your brain to stimulate the release of all that lovely cocktail of hormones, and encourages your labour to progress smoothly. Without this pressure, labour is often something of a stop–start affair.

4) LESS PAINFUL

As well as making your contractions more efficient, being upright is also less painful: research has shown, unequivocally, that active births require less pain relief.[15] Moving helps to alleviate discomfort – in fact, in my yoga for pregnancy classes we spend a lot of time on all fours, doing pelvic rotations and noting how different movements can alleviate discomfort in different parts of the pelvis and back. The women in my classes very often report back that they subsequently spent a lot of their labours on all fours and that moving through contractions really helped reduce their pain.

Being upright stops the uterus from having to work harder than it needs to. The uterus is basically a very large muscle. The harder the muscle works, the more painful it is. (Think about your thighs when you run or biceps when you lift – the harder they work, the more you feel it.) It is the same with the uterus. During a contraction the uterus naturally tilts forwards. If you are lying down, the energy required for this forward tilting is significantly increased. The result is that the uterus will have to work harder, and the more exertion, the more pain. One woman recently confided in me, 'I am not afraid of birth. My only worry is that my mother said the whole way through her labour with me she had a desperate urge to get on her knees. The midwives made her lie on her back, but all she wanted to do was get up and lean forwards. She said having to lie down almost drove her crazy. I am just worried that the same thing might happen to me.' If she was made to give birth lying down, then her fears would have been realised, as most women feel an instinctive urge to get up. Luckily, in this particular instance the mother in question was cared for by a fabulous midwife, who was a huge advocate of active birth. She moved around, overnight, for a total of nine hours before giving birth to a very healthy baby girl of 7 lb 6 oz, having spent most of her labour on her hands and knees!

5) LESS CHANCE OF FOETAL DISTRESS

Giving birth actively is also fundamentally safer for your baby. One of the most commonly cited reasons for an emergency Caesarean is that a baby is in distress. If you ask a woman what position she was in when foetal distress was diagnosed, she will usually tell you it was on her back. Yet most women will also tell you that during late pregnancy they can no longer sleep on their backs. Even if it is not too uncomfortable to do so, they will say it instinctively doesn't feel right. And as is often the case during pregnancy, your instincts are often a very wise guide.

By the ninth month of pregnancy your belly, including the baby, placenta and amniotic fluid is a minimum of 20 lb – the equivalent to no less than a very large hessian sack of potatoes. When lying down, this weight rests on your major arteries, which run from your heart to the placenta and back again.[16] The large artery of the heart (the descending aorta) hinders circulation to the uterus and placenta, which can result in the baby lacking oxygen. The large veins that lead to the heart (the inferior vena cava) restricts the returning blood flow and can lead to hypertension in the mother, and to other circulatory problems that can cause much heavier bleeding after birth. Get up and there is no such compression, and so none of these avoidable complications. (And if you did have them, you at least know it was something other than your position that caused them.) It is probably a grim truth that there has been many a woman who has undergone a Caesarean – major abdominal surgery – when a simple change of position would have sufficed.

Securing Yourself an Active Birth

Rather wonderfully, a lot of the work has been done for you. Whereas in the 1970s and '80s mothers practically had to petition to get off their backs, knowledge of the benefits of being active in labour means it is becoming more mainstream. It's been almost 20 years since the National Childbirth Trust (NCT), the biggest providers of antenatal care in the UK, introduced a section on being mobile in labour and created a worksheet of possible positions a woman might consider adopting. More and more midwives and doctors are familiar with the research and many actively encourage movement throughout labour. But the practice is still not as widespread as it should be, despite science being on a woman's side. Many hospitals, for example, are happy to allow you the freedom to move during the first stage of labour, but still might require you to lie down and put your feet in stirrups to birth your baby. If you find yourself in this position (pardon the pun!), yet would actually like to remain active for the second stage, too, you are well within your rights to question your birth attendant. Research has shown that the benefits of being active do not simply apply to the first stage. There are additional benefits in the second stage, too: contractions tend to be more powerful, which means the expulsion reflex is more effective; the angle of the baby's descent and the space in the pelvis is optimised and, once again, being upright will harness gravity to good effect. As hard as it is to try to find a voice during labour itself, it is essential to speak up if you are very uncomfortable with something. At the very least ask for an explanation or get your partner to.

If you are now suitably convinced that being active during labour and birth is a good idea, then you'll need to get yourself physically and mentally prepared. Our culture is a relatively sedentary one. Many of us sit down for most of the day, shuttling from the breakfast table, to the car, to the office and back to the sofa with only moderate movement in between. Compared to our Far Eastern counterparts, we tend to be limited in the positions we routinely adopt; sitting cross-legged is uncomfortable for many and squatting often impossible. Travelling in Asia, you see many people by roadside stalls, eating their meals while perched comfortably in a deep squat, yet this would be an unthinkable dining option for a lot of us.

So we need to get moving. Once you are familiar with the positions that you might want to adopt for labour and birth, it is important to accustom your body to them. This is an integral part of yoga for pregnancy classes, so it is advisable to attend a class if possible. If you start early, the positions will seep into your muscles and your mindset and become so familiar that by the time you come to give birth you will consider them to be part of your own repertoire. You will also find that, over the weeks, you become more flexible, better aligned and stronger despite your growing baby and belly. An alternative to a class is regular yoga practice at home that includes active birthing positions. (Though again clearance from your midwife before throwing yourself into yoga unguided and, at the very least, use a DVD.

It is essential that your birth partner is familiar with the positions you want to use in labour and birth. Unless he is unusually keen and has read up on the whole birth experience, the chances are he will have been brainwashed into thinking that it is normal for a woman to labour on her back. While the raw science behind the idea of being mobile in labour means that fathers are not hard to convince, it is essential that whoever is supporting you does not react strangely to you adopting primal positions. I have heard it said far too many times that a woman felt desperate to move during labour, but was so concerned about how her husband might react that she endured immobility against her better judgement. Birth is primal and animal, and your movements and positions should reflect this – make sure your partner is prepared for anything!

Active Birth Positions

Below is a series of possible birth positions. There are many and countless variations of each one – none are prescriptive. They are illustrated as examples, as the idea is to simply move as your instincts compel you to, free from misconceptions or inhibitions. It is also essential not to adopt any position that feels uncomfortable, nor feel a compulsion to move all the time. Many women labour in an upright or semi-upright position but in fact move very little, and often less and less over the course of their labour, moaning and rocking and moving backwards and forwards, but staying very much in one little private corner rather than pacing anywhere in particular. The main thing is to heed your own inclinations and be uninhibited mentally and physically.

POSITIONS FOR THE FIRST STAGE

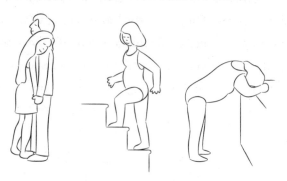

Being upright enables you to rotate your hips and use gravity to assist the descent of your baby.

In very early labour, standing, walking, being upright and leaning against someone or something are all good. Going up and down the stairs can also be a useful way of getting labour going and getting the baby into the optimum position.

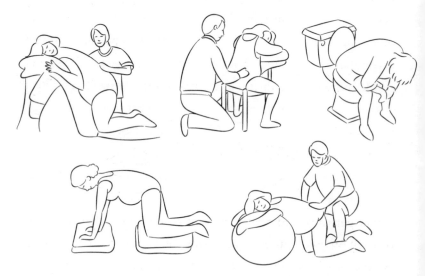

Positions, like the ones above, where you are leaning forward are also effective. They are easier to sustain, make your sacrum and back easily available for massage and effective counter-pressure, and really open the pelvis. You can either kneel or use furniture – beds, chairs and beanbags – as useful props.

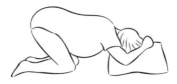

In the case of an unexpectedly fast labour, you can use the knee–chest position (above) to slow things down. This is also a good position to use if you know your baby is posterior (back-to-back – see chapter six for full explanation) as it gives the baby room to spiral around. Finally, if you have an anterior lip (part of the cervix that is not quite fully dilated at the onset of stage two), then you will often be advised to get into this position to pant rather than push through your contractions. This gives the cervix a little more time to dilate fully without unduly swelling.

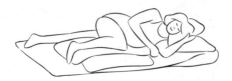

If you get tired and really do want to lie down, then position yourself on your left-hand side, with your upper body supported by cushions. This will give your sacrum the freedom to move and there is no danger of compressing the major arteries to and from the heart.

POSITIONS FOR THE SECOND STAGE

Again, don't think of these positions as prescriptive; they are options depending on how you are feeling and what your midwife advises.

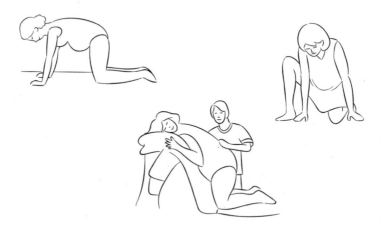

In these positions, you can feel the weight of the ground beneath you and it will give you something to push against.

You can either sit, kneel or use furniture – beds, chairs and beanbags.

Sitting on something – a birth stool or someone's lap, for example – can also be a good position for the second stage as it helps to really focus your energies down and into your bottom.

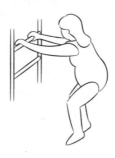

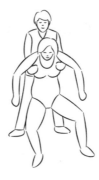

An upright or supported squat also enables the pelvis to open to its maximum, but as these positions get very tiring you will need to be well supported.

The Other Side of Active Birth

The physical side of active birth is only half the story. Although upright and mobile positions are key, a truly active birth is also about being at the centre of your own birth experience, active in its preparation and in the process of birth as it unfolds. All too often it is the medical establishment that takes control and we defer to its authority. Sometimes you might be grateful for medical staff taking over, but all too often mothers feel robbed. As a midwife in the American film *The Business of Being Born* says, 'Women don't need to be rescued from their own birth, they need to lay claim to their experience.' [17]

Obstetric intervention in birth has saved lives, but its value as a safety net does not justify its routine use in low-risk birth, or its having given rise to protocols that take the place of a woman's own desires or instincts. Under normal conditions a woman is best left to be her own director, behaving in an instinctive and, importantly, uninhibited way. For many of us, however, this is easier said than done. Medicine teaches intervention, and we are not very good at saying no. Research into our relationship with 'authority' was conducted on the London underground: in a series of experiments, volunteers went on to tube carriages and asked people to give up their seats. Initially the volunteers were dressed in normal, everyday clothes. When they were, only 55 per cent of people willingly stood up or moved to another seat to allow the volunteer to sit down. The experiment was then repeated, but this time the volunteers wore uniforms of different types – some were dressed as soldiers, others as doctors, others as policemen. This time, when people were asked to give up their seats, there was *100 per cent* compliance! We don't dare, it seems, to challenge the uniform.

Doctors do not need to have seen this study to know how much power they wield. And while most do not abuse our trust, many advocate hospital protocol without being able to say why. The use of Electronic Foetal Monitors (EFMs) is a case in point. These monitors record the baby's heart rate alongside uterine pressure, displaying the results on a screen. The most commonly used are external ones, which consist of two belts attached around the mother's belly. The lower one picks up the baby's heart rate by ultrasound, in the same way as the hand-held Doppler used in antenatal visits or at home births. The upper belt picks up contractions. Research has shown conclusively that Electronic Foetal Monitoring bestows no benefits on the baby or the mother, but instead increases the chances of a Caesarean delivery. My advice is that in all but complicated situations, request an alternative or at the very least a mobile option. Thankfully, hospitals are increasingly trying to comply with the new NICE guidelines and are monitoring intermittently unless they absolutely deem it necessary to do otherwise.

It is difficult under any circumstances to question what is presented as a necessary procedure and protocol, and especially so when there is a baby in the mix. Many women understandably accept what is done to them as being necessary, but if you are in any doubt, no harm can come from questioning. A father in one of my recent workshops suggested that couples ask the question 'How necessary is this?' when faced with any intervention.

Remember, in most cases you have time on your side. Ask as many questions as you feel you need to about what the intervention is, why it is being proposed and its possible downsides. Try not to rush, or allow yourself to be rushed. If you find yourself becoming frustrated, then take a deep breath and calmly ask everything you feel you need to know. In extreme cases, you could ask if you and your partner could have a few moments to talk about things alone.

A good option is to ask if 'waiting and watching' is possible. In other words, asking if you can continue without intervention – if that is what you want – for a specific period, so long as the baby is being monitored and continues to be okay.

Another option – and one which mothers find useful because they say it stops them from sounding simply defiant – is to suggest that you try a simpler, less invasive option first. So for example, if your midwife is clock-watching and is itching to speed things up with artificial oxytocin, then you could suggest that you and your partner go for a walk, change your position or increase your energy levels with a small snack or a teaspoon of honey. As a wonderful midwife by the name of Naomi Morton always says, 'Try hugs before drugs.' Often these simple measures work wonders, and if they don't, then at least in your own mind you know you've tried.

You could be forgiven for assuming that hospital protocols are based on perfect science, yet time and again they have been found to be lacking. Don't just assume that because it is hospital policy it makes scientific sense. They are only based on guidelines and they can be flexible. Time limits on stages of labour are often arbitrary and protocols can be wildly different from hospital to hospital. Getting a copy of the hospital's policy notes in advance can be useful, as it will give you your parameters. It is also good to know your own rights as well. I am not keen on getting everyone to turn their birth into a miniature revolution, but if you know that you are going to a large teaching hospital with fairly rigid protocols, then knowing what you can and can't expect in advance is probably useful. The AIMS (see page 268) booklet 'Am I Allowed?' makes good reading in this regard. Whatever happens, if on the day something is being advocated that you or your partner are not sure about, then you are well within your rights to ask. Remember it is your birth and your baby. There is never any harm in a simple question.

In fact, being informed should be the lynchpin of all that you do in your birth preparation. As Lucy Atkins says in the fantastic book *Blooming Birth*, a lot of us take more time over our summer holiday plans than we do over our births.[18] A generation ago women had no excuse. There were very few books, no classes and so most went through the system, ended up on their backs, legs splayed, drugged up to the eyeballs. And that is where our birth stories come from. We, however, are in an altogether different position. We can educate ourselves, we have options, we have choices. Find out all you can about birth – read this book, and then try to make your way through my 'desert island' suggestions (see page 267). Sign up to an antenatal class, but do your homework. There are classes and then there are classes. Ask around for local recommendations, as often a good class has more to do with the teacher than the particular brand of birth she teaches. Remember, it is very difficult to find your voice in labour if you haven't found it beforehand. It is inaccurate to suggest you will always be in control – in fact, the whole point is you need to be able to let go, to lose control, but you want to do it while still remaining very much at the centre of your own experience. Preparing beforehand will help keep you there.

Make sure you prepare yourself physically. Active Births are physically strenuous so you will need to be fit, strong and healthy. Eat well and exercise gently. Seek out aquanatal, pregnancy yoga or Pilates classes. The aim is not to become a fitness fanatic, but to keep your body supple and your muscles toned (even if they look like they are dissolving before your very eyes!) And make sure that you also use your pregnancy to re-educate yourself in the art of relaxation – any good birth class will incorporate it. Alternatively, get hold of some Natal Hypnotherapy CDs and treat yourself to a daily half-hour of relaxing. A birth is so, so much better if you can relax into it and through it. It might seem a tall order from where you are sitting, but I assure you it is possible.

Whatever you do, make decisions about your birth – the who's, the how's and the where's – wisely and with conviction.

A useful starting point for feeling at the centre of your own experience is to write a birth plan. Sceptics argue that birth plans set up unrealistic expectations on the part of the mother, but so long as you remain open to possibility and change, they are a fantastic opportunity to order your thoughts and to work out what it is you are hoping for. And writing down your aspirations increases the chances of them happening. A now infamous study dubbed the 'Harvard' study tried to prove to us that writing down your goals increased the chance of you achieving them. But it was infamous, because it didn't actually happen! Though the study was obviously meaningless, it has prompted other real but less-publicised studies that show that writing something down and committing to it makes a material difference.[19] If nothing else, it is an act of assertiveness and a commitment to taking matters, as much as possible, into your own hands.

Obviously, there is an element of the unknown involved in every birth experience. Assuming that you can write down what you want and then get it would of course be unrealistic. But it is equally inaccurate to suggest that the outcome of every birth is pure chance. Planning for your labour while remaining open to change is the best way to maximise your chances of a positive experience. Writing down what you would like and then discussing it with both your partner and midwife can be an important, even an essential, part of the process of approaching birth in an empowered way. It gives you the opportunity to work out what really matters to you, and to tackle any fears you might have head-on. It also means that you and the people who are looking after you are on the same page, quite literally. As one of the women in my class suggested, birth plans are a way of giving a midwife you may never have met a flavour of what sort of birth you are after.

Your birth plan needs to cover the simple things: where you want to be and who you want with you, as well as your preferences regarding pain relief, monitoring, vaginal examinations, the possible use of water and being active. Some birth plan templates also stipulate preferences over intervention, though I think this is futile. The truth is, no one is going to ask for a forceps delivery, but if it came down to it and the hospital said it was your only option, then would you argue that it wasn't on your birth plan? By all means if there is anything that truly frightens you, make sure you write that down but otherwise try to keep your plan about what you would like rather than what you wouldn't. And keep it short. No one is going to read and absorb a plan that extends to three pages. One side of A4 and you have a good chance that anyone looking after you will know what you would, in an ideal world, like. See the box (below) for ideas about what to include.

BIRTH PLAN TEMPLATE

- Your name.
- Your partner's name and telephone number.
- Contact details for anyone else who will support you – this should include your doula if you have one, or anyone

---

else who will be at the birth with you, as well as the babysitter's telephone numbers if you have other children who need to be looked after.

- The telephone number and address of the hospital you are giving birth at, or the midwife's number if you are going to be at home.

- A general description of the type of birth you want: for example, you're very keen to have a natural birth or you're adamant that you want an epidural; you're happy to see how it goes on the day. You could almost think of this as your 'twitter' version, your 140-word ideal birth.

- Any specific and pressing issues or fears: it is important to state anything in particular that you are worried about so that it can be addressed. It might be that you are nervous of being naked, or that you don't want additional people around unless absolutely necessary, or that you have a particular worry about tearing. If this is your second birth, feel free to state things about your first birth that might have unnerved or upset you.

- The environment and atmosphere: think about all the things that would make you most comfortable and relaxed and specify what you'd like. Go back to chapter one to work out what sorts of things you might want to consider. If you especially like a particular smell or oil then write it down in your birth plan.

- What you'd like for pain relief: it might be nothing at all or you might be determined to have the smorgasbord. It's up to you, but write it down. Remember, even if you request an epidural there will be quite a bit of time during labour that you'll do without it, so consider what you might want up until that point. This is the place to talk about water if you'd like to use it. If there is anything you'd specifically like to avoid then say that too: for example, some women are keen on the TENS machine, others aren't, or some mothers might like gas and air but no pethidine. If you don't want to be offered pain relief but would rather be left to ask for it, then write that down as well.

- Active birth positions: you won't be able to state in advance which specific positions you will want to use; that will happen instinctively on the day and be based partly on trial and error. It also changes throughout labour. But specify in your Birth plan if you categorically don't want to be on your back.

- Interventions and their alternatives: this can help to jog your own and your partner's memory on the day. Specify if there are any interventions that you would like to avoid – for example induction, Electronic Foetal Monitoring, oxytocin drip, vaginal examinations – and what you'd like to try in their place, if it comes to that.

- When the baby is born: would you like the baby to be passed to you, or to your partner? If skin-to-skin contact is important to you, then write that down, as well as whether you would prefer a managed or natural third stage (see page 176 before you fill in this bit!)

Obviously it's impossible to be completely comprehensive with a template, and you won't be able to write it all down in one sitting. Think of it as a work in progress, though one that might need some editing at the end. You might want photos, you might not. You might need someone to close the door on overzealous relatives until you are ready for them. The specifics of your birth and your preferences for it will be yours alone. Keep a little book or a scrap of paper with you in your handbag, so you can write things down as and when you think of them, and then you can add them to your master copy later. Remember, as with births, there are endless permutations of the birth plan.

Do not assume that your birth will follow your plan to the letter. And be prepared to be flexible on the day. Your birth can still be a really positive experience even when it diverges dramatically from your plan. In fact the process of thinking about it, and writing it down, and talking about it with your birth partner is far more important than the final plan itself.

In a world of managed births and high intervention, an active birth might seem revolutionary but it is far from new. When women are left to labour in the way that they wish, they almost always choose to be active – to move and to feel that they are in control of their experience. A woman's perception of her birth is often less about whether she ended up with an epidural or a caesarean and more about how empowered and involved she felt. While for many a modern woman, the experience of birth has been a disappointing one, recent history has shown that with understanding and wilfulness, many a woman has been able to secure herself an active birth. And while being active does not guarantee you a natural birth, it significantly improves your chances.

SUMMARY

- All over the world and since the beginning of time, women have laboured instinctively in upright positions.

- Being active will make your labour quicker and less painful, as well as reduce your need for intervention.

- An active labour is safer for the baby as there is less chance of foetal distress.

- Practise active birth positions in the context of a yoga class if you can get to one, otherwise do simple exercises at home. The main aim is to be mentally and physically prepared to be upright and mobile during labour.

- Remember that the positions are not prescriptive. It is essential that you follow your instincts and labour in whatever positions come naturally.

- Make sure your partner understands the benefits of active birth positions and is familiar with what they might look like.

- An active birth is not just about moving, but about being at the centre of your own birth experience. At all times remember that it is your baby and your birth.

- Read up as much as you can and get yourself to an antenatal class, preferably one that has been recommended as some are better than others.

- Know your rights by reading the AIMS (see page 268) booklet 'Am I Allowed?' and speak up if something is being advocated that you don't feel comfortable with.

CHAPTER 3

Support During Labour
The Dolphin Ring

'If doulas were a drug it would be unethical not to use them.'
Marshall Klaus

Birth is a mammoth act of letting go, both physically and mentally. On the physical side, the cervix is a sphincter and an extraordinary one at that. It needs to have the strength to keep what eventually becomes 22 lb of baby, placenta and amniotic fluid inside, but then, when the time comes, it needs to have the capacity to thin and soften and open up a full 10 cm. Look at 10 cm on a ruler – it's probably wider than you think. When you think about it, this is really quite amazing. No other sphincter in your body is capable of quite such dramatic gymnastics. To say the body needs to let go is arguably something of an understatement.

And then, of course, there is the whole mental side of letting go that we looked at in the first chapter. That softening of the mind, allowing yourself to be vulnerable and, crucially, switching off your chattering brain so that you can retreat into the primal brain.

It is not an oversimplification to say that to let go physically and mentally you need to completely relax. And a key part of this, in addition to the atmosphere you create and the practice you do throughout your pregnancy, is the support you have. To relax fully and deeply, it is essential that you feel safe, secure and emotionally nurtured.

In an ideal world everyone would have one-to-one midwifery care, in which you get to know your midwife throughout your pregnancy and build up a relationship and a rapport that would feed positively into your labour. Traditionally, that was how women were cared for – initially, quite informally, by mothers, grandmothers, friends and neighbours, and then gradually by midwives as the role became a more formal one. And up until relatively recently, midwives were greatly esteemed in the community, forming the lynchpin of women's lives. As Tina Cassidy aptly says in her book *Birth: A History*, one would assume that given our long dependence on midwives, such women would still reign today. Yet, increasingly, women are being attended to by obstetricians, and where midwifery still prevails the workload is so enormous that the emotional side of a midwife's job has all but been scheduled out of existence. Usually women are assigned a team of midwives for their antenatal care, and only the lucky ones come across one of the midwives from her team during labour and birth itself.

Staff shortages have led to even the most well-meaning midwife having to attend several births at once. One study reported that a low-risk mother having her first baby in a teaching hospital was attended to by *16* different people, and yet she was still left alone most of the time. Another study found that women giving birth in hospital encountered an average of six unfamiliar professionals during labour, with some at the extreme reporting up to 14 different attendants.[20] All too often, women complain of having been hooked up to a hospital monitor and then ignored. It is not uncommon for midwives to come and go with alarming frequency, and, worse still, to make very limited eye contact, if at all, when they are in the room. Yet, interestingly, women very often judge their birth experience on the quality of emotional care they are given. One elated mother wrote to me after the birth of her second daughter, emphasising again and again how wonderful it had been because – wait for it … drum roll – the midwives had actually listened to her. That is it. As simple as that. Nothing extraordinary, nothing amazing that technology delivered, but a better birth because someone actually cared.

And this woman is not the only person whose experience was enhanced dramatically by good emotional nurture and support. In 2007 a huge review was undertaken, bringing together all the available research on the impact of continuous support in labour. The review was in response to the rising concern that women were – as the studies suggested – increasingly being left to labour alone, at best attended to by a stream of different people and at worst by machines, their output designed to take the place of a midwife's nurturing hand. The research was extensive to say the least – it covered 16 separate trials, across 11 countries, and included almost 13,500 women. The results of the review were unequivocal. Women who were continuously supported throughout their labour had dramatically fewer Caesarean sections – up to 50 per cent less, far fewer forceps or vacuum extractions, and much less need for epidural anaesthesia and other forms of pain relief. Mothers also said that they felt much happier about their birth experience. And the positive results did not end there. All of the described benefits were increased even further when the support for the woman was not linked to the hospital she was in, and when it began early on in labour.[21]

In a world besieged by medical technology and complex innovation and where intervention in the birth process is now the norm, the message could not be more clear. *The simple but continuous presence of a support person in the room, a completely non-invasive alternative, is one of the most effective ways to improve birth outcome and experience.*

So Who Will Support You?

MIDWIVES

In some parts of the UK – and it really is a postcode lottery – one-to-one midwifery is alive and well. Ask whether it is available in your area, and if it is not, whether there is a midwife-led unit or birthing centre option (see page 25) as an alternative. While these places don't always offer individualised care in the antenatal period, they are usually housed by smaller teams of midwives, so you might well have at least met the person you end up labouring with and in all likelihood she will only have you to look after when you are giving birth. The midwives in these places tend to be less busy than hospital midwives, so are more capable of attending to the emotional side of labour and birth.

If knowing who will be there is something that really resonates with you, and you want to be absolutely sure of it, then an independent midwife is another option. They are not cheap (a package of care usually costs between £2,000 and £4,500), but usually provide fantastic support and care antenatally, throughout labour and postnatally. They are effectively freelance or private midwives, fully trained by the Nursing Midwifery Council but working independently. Some will do hospital births, depending on what their contract allows, while others just do home births. Find out what they are able to do in the early interview stages. It is also, I believe, important to shop around and make sure that you have a good immediate rapport with your midwife and that you trust her judgement. Ask questions that will give you a feel for her way of thinking; what she would do in an emergency, what she might suggest as pain relief, what her own experience of birth has been.

Whatever care you choose, remember that the vast majority of midwives do the job because they are passionate about looking after women in labour, and there are gems scattered all over the country, working hard in even the largest of hospitals.

DADS

In addition to your main carer, it is important to consider who else will be with you for the birth. Not so long ago, your baby's father wasn't really a birth partner option. His allocated spot was propping up the bar at the pub, stressfully gulping down pints, with a mandatory cigar at the ready for the good news. The closest he ever got to the action was pacing the corridors of the hospital, straining to hear sounds of his baby's arrival. Only 50 years ago it was almost unheard of for a man to be with his wife or partner during labour. Fast-forward a mere half a century and now almost all partners are ringside. At last count, 96 per cent of fathers attended the birth of their children in the UK. Celebrities are applauded for leaving key tournaments or for shunning film schedules to be by their wife's side and more often than not it is the father who emerges triumphantly from the hospital with babe in arms. Antenatal classes for couples are now big business, and some teachers proclaim the thirst for knowledge of fathers is now so extreme, that they are starting to run dedicated workshops for dads. Fathers are not only at the births of their children, but are often active participants, breathing along with the mother, physically holding her, cutting the umbilical cord and filling water pools – in some cases, everything bar the act of labour itself.

For some women, this is exactly how it should be. Many would not consider giving birth without their partners – such was the amazingly calming presence mine maintained throughout my birth experiences, I threatened to hire him out as a birth partner!

But among all of this razzamatazz and cultural expectation is very often a dazed, confused and even terrified father, unsure of his role. And whether he should be there at all is the subject of some debate. Michel Odent, the French obstetrician-turned-midwife and an ardent proponent of natural birth, suggests that some men can be misplaced in the birth room. He argues that far from being a help to a labouring mother, the father can actually be a hindrance, making a labour longer or more difficult than it needs to be. While some accuse Odent of sacrilege, to spark debate in this field is entirely healthy. I have had many women confess to me that they felt entirely uncomfortable about their partner being there, but were afraid to say anything in case they hurt his feelings or made themselves virtual social outcasts by bucking the trend. Debate and, crucially, communication between couples is essential. Birth practice is not always good practice, and as compelling as social pressure might be, it has never been a good reason to do anything.

It is essential that you ask yourself two questions:

Does he want to be there?

Most will want to be. Being privy to the birth of your own child is an extraordinary event, and most dads wouldn't want to miss it for the world. But, understandably, some fathers are not sure how they will feel with the enormity of the experience, or with the potential stress entailed in watching their wife or partner go through labour. This doesn't make them bad fathers. It in no way means that they aren't dedicated to the cause. It simply means that they are not comfortable with the responsibility that comes with being a birth partner. And a reticent or, even worse, fearful observer to the proceedings is the very father that Michel Odent is concerned about. Fear is contagious, so much so that American military researchers are actually trying to harness it as a weapon of war. If your husband or partner is fearful, it is highly likely that you will be, too, and adrenaline – the hormone produced in response to fear – is a direct impediment to the first stage of labour.

Do you want him there?

And even more pertinently, will you be able to truly let go in front of him? What I call the litmus test for this is an admittedly base but amusing little question: can you do 'number twos' in front of your partner? If the answer is yes, then he should stay in the running for birth partner. If the answer is a resounding no, then without guilt or worry, you should think about considering someone else to be by your side. And the reason for this is very simple. As we saw in chapter one, to labour safely and easily you need, above all, to be able to switch off your front brain (see page 13). For that you need a conducive environment, a sense of being protected and the capacity to completely let go and become entirely primal. For some women, this letting go is completely plausible with their partner or husband in the room. They have a no-holds-barred, all-hang-out relationship where nothing is taboo. For them, he is a source of security, and having him there means feeling safer and more able to let go. For others, their relationship is characterised by the maintenance of a certain mystery. Some things – including bodily functions – are kept behind closed doors.

A very close friend of mine, who is of the ardent belief that her husband's presence at her first birth was the very reason she couldn't let go and ended up having a Caesarean, also confessed that for the first seven years of their marriage she successfully maintained the illusion that she never, ever farted! If this sounds like your relationship, consider carefully how you might be willing to behave, or not, with your partner there and make plans accordingly. It might not be the case that your partner needs to disappear completely, but maybe just that you have someone else there too so that you can be flexible on the day.

APART FROM DADS

I am well aware that not all babies are born into families with fathers around. Many women are having babies as single mothers, and there are, of course, increasing numbers of same-sex parents out there. If you fall into that camp, then you are by no means forgotten. If your baby's father is not around, you can still consider who your birth partner can and should be in exactly the same way. It is important that you are supported, and that the person who supports you is someone you trust and can let go in front of. That person's role will be the same as any father's would be, so the decision-making process is exactly the same, as is the part he or she can play in the birth room.

The Father's Role in the Birth Room

Assuming that you have now asked yourselves all the right questions, and dad is going to be there during labour and birth, you need to decide on his role. In Ray Mears' *Bushcraft Survival* series there is a wonderful scene where Mears explores the versatility of the Baobab tree to the Hadza tribe. They eat its fruits, dig for its roots, use its leaves and bark – and, amazingly, the women of the tribe give birth in the hollowed-out trunk of the tree itself.

In fact, entire generations of the same village have been born in the very same place. When a father asks me how he should consider his role, I liken it to being that very tree. The best role for a father to play is that which usually comes naturally to him. To act as the protector, creating a safe place in which his partner can birth.

With this in mind, I am going to address fathers directly in the next section. Get them to read chapter one and then this bit, at the very least!

THE GUARDIAN OF THE ENVIRONMENT

In practical terms, you can ensure that the environment is conducive to labour – turn down the lights and question the presence of all but the most necessary people. You should ask yourself the question 'Could I sleep in here?', and, if you couldn't, alter the environment in whatever way seems feasible. Dim lighting, privacy and the ability to move and behave instinctively all make a dramatic difference to a woman during labour. Remember, also, that less is more. Sometimes saying nothing is the best support you can give, and the perfect way to allow your partner to switch off and retreat into the back of her brain. It is therefore essential to understand the physiology of birth and the mechanics of the brain during the birth process. An understanding of transition and the normality of a woman's often inexplicable behaviour at this point will also help you to stay calm yourself and guide you to say the right things.

THE ADVOCATE

If necessary, you might find the need to be a buffer between your partner and the medical system. Women in labour very often need an advocate. I once spoke to a woman who somewhat unconventionally had asked her own father to be her birth partner when her second child was born. Her decision was met with raised eyebrows by some and many people admitted that they thought it was wholly inappropriate. But to the woman herself, it made perfect sense. She said, 'During my first birth experience I felt what I had lacked was an advocate. Throughout my life, my father has always fought for me, so he seemed an obvious choice second time around.'

Many mothers feel strongly about the birth experience they would like but, like most of us, lose their nerve in the face of a forthright doctor. As we saw in the London underground experiment (see page 50), in the face of authority all but the seriously stubborn tend to cower. Add to the mix the vulnerability that women feel during labour and the heady cocktail of hormones coursing through their veins, and disagreeing with hospital policy becomes even more difficult. This is where an informed birth partner can play a crucial role, speaking up for a woman as and when is necessary.

BEING RESPONSIVE

It is essential that in the same way that mothers need to be open and willing to a change in circumstances, so too should fathers. Plans to massage or give physical support throughout labour are good, but be prepared that your partner's needs might change and often on a dime. Responding to her needs is important, but so too is flexibility. One poor hapless father, whose wife had insisted on being massaged throughout her entire first labour, found himself shouted away when he attempted the same loving touch second time around. That time, she wanted to be left completely alone. Man is an unpredictable beast, and a woman in labour even more so.

It is also important to be ready to offer up physical support when it is necessary. An active birth is hard work and very often a mother, particularly in the second stage, will need someone to lean on, pull against or hold on to. Fathers can really come into their own in this regard, providing much needed physical support and intimacy that would be harder for a stranger.

LOOKING AFTER YOURSELF

Don't forget your own needs. Becoming a father, for the first, second, third or even fourth time, is a wholly emotional experience and can give rise to a whole host of feelings, concerns and, very commonly, an increasing sense of responsibility. During the birth itself, it is essential to keep your energy levels up, stay hydrated, have a break if you need to and, if at all possible, pass the baton to someone else for short periods if the labour is long. Before and after the birth, find people to talk to. I read a staggering statistic that the incidence of male postnatal depression is as high as 10 per cent. It is not unusual for a man to feel confused, rejected, exhausted or under pressure, even if he is also elated at the birth of his child. It is a gross generalisation to say that women tend to talk about their feelings, whereas men bottle things up, but it is often the case that men don't say what is on their mind. If this applies to you, find a means of release – even if it is going for a beer or playing a game of squash rather than having a heart-to-heart. There is increasing and welcome acknowledgement that we do not nurture our mothers enough in this society, but it is also the case that fathers have few outlets, too. I have added some contacts at the end of the book for mothers, but also include some for fathers (see page 269). For a family to function happily as a whole, everyone needs to be looked after: father, mother and baby.

PRACTICAL JOBS FOR DAD

- Make sure you know the way to the hospital and an alternative route if traffic is likely to be an issue. Build a nest of cushions on the back seat for your partner to lean over. Drive much more slowly than you think you need to and come to a virtual standstill at speed bumps.

- Make sure the petrol tank is full, and that the baby seat and the hospital bag are in the car. You won't be allowed to leave the hospital with your newborn unless you have an appropriate seat.

- Remember your wallet, keys, camera and phone. It sounds patronising (or annoyingly mother-like) but in the heat of labour it is very easy to forget simple things!

- Offer your partner lower-back massages or counter-pressure on her sacrum, and do so between contractions. In fact, anything you do, be it touch or talk, do it between contractions. During a contraction leave her be and let her retreat.

- Offer her sips of water, lukewarm, sugary tea and the occasional light snack. A spoonful of honey can also be nice. Mothers tend not to want to eat or drink much in labour, so if her energy seems to be waning you might have to convince her it's a good idea.

- Remind her to breathe. If she seems to be unresponsive and is holding her breath, simply breathe deeply with her. You'll find she quickly locks in with you.

- Be prepared for birth to be messy – your partner might throw up, poo and her waters might break all over your shoes. When your baby is born, it will in all likelihood be covered in vernix (see page 171). In advance this all sounds a bit icky, but in the heat of the moment none of it will matter as much as you think it will. The midwife is so used to it that she won't even flinch. It's important that you don't either.

Doulas

If the father of your child is not going to be with you, or if you feel that you and your husband or partner would like a bit more support, then a doula is a fantastic and increasingly popular option. While they are more than happy to be your sole support, more often than not doulas work alongside you and your partner, supporting you both through your birth preparation, labour and sometimes into the immediate postnatal period. 'I have two hands, so figured I would need two people to hold them' was how one mother described her decision to have a doula on board.

Often after a birth it is fathers who wax lyrical about the doula. Not only are they aware of the visible reassurance that a doula provides their wife or partner before the birth and in labour, but they very often say that they too felt reassured having someone knowledgeable and calm by their side from start to finish. And their delight should come as no surprise. Births with doulas have 50 per cent fewer Caesareans, 40 per cent fewer assisted deliveries, less use of pain relief, and are considered more positive experiences by the mother. As an added bonus, postnatal depression is less likely after having given birth with the support of a doula.

Named after the Greek for female slave, because she was traditionally privileged to attend to the mistress of the house, doulas are there to entirely care for the emotional and physical needs of the mother and her family during labour. They are not intended to replace the midwife, and are not medically trained, though many have been on training programmes and all have a fundamental understanding of the physiology of birth.

Sometimes all that is necessary is for the doula to simply be there – a constant and reassuring presence – but she can also take a much more active role, depending on what you might want and what circumstances dictate. Obviously all doulas are different but generally she will:

- Teach both you and your partner about birth.
- Help you explore and process any worries or fears you have about birth, or any lingering concerns about a previous birth.
- Be available as a source of reassurance and support – via both phone and email – leading up to the birth. In fact, one woman said that the best thing about having a doula was to have a source of reassurance on speed dial!
- Advise you if you are overdue.
- Come to you when you feel you need support during labour.
- Be with you all the way through labour regardless of its duration.
- Enable your partner to take on board whatever role he feels comfortable with, explain medical terms or procedures if necessary and give him the chance to have tea breaks or rests if the labour is long. A doula will not get in the way – good doulas are sensitive to the enormity of birth within a family.
- Come to see you after the birth to talk it through and celebrate your baby with you.

A doula's role during the labour itself can also include advocacy, massage, gentle encouragement, guidance with breathing, reassurance or help in changing positions. It might also be more practical help that is needed – baking muffins with a mother's other children while she labours at home, making tea for everyone or keeping a birth pool filled with warm water. To be honest, the intricacies of the doula's role matter less than the fact that you can be absolutely assured that she will be with you from the very beginning to the very end, no matter what. As a student of mine recently testified, 'It wasn't so much what the doula did that made the difference,' she said, 'but rather that she was there for the whole time.'

Another woman told me quite enthusiastically, 'I am absolutely convinced that I would not have been able to get through the more difficult parts of my birth if it wasn't for my doula holding my hand. She said almost nothing, but whenever I was worried I would instinctively look to her for reassurance, and because she looked calm, I stayed calm.'

In fact, the experience of women with doulas is so overwhelmingly positive that almost all the women who have had one proclaim they would never give birth without one. And societies in which women speak of little or no pain in childbirth (and believe it or not they do exist) are also the ones where mothers are well nurtured by other women, before, during and after their labours.

FIVE REASONS WHY DADS LIKE HAVING DOULAS

1 A doula will be there from start to finish no matter what, which means you can rest, get a breath of fresh air, and make tea without worrying that your partner is ever alone.
2 A doula will know what you were meant to have learned in your childbirth class, but now can't remember.
3 A doula will know what questions to ask.
4 A doula will understand birth terminology and be able to explain it to you.
5 A doula will keep you, and your partner, calm.

THE DOULA PACKAGE

Most doulas offer a standard package consisting of two or three antenatal meetings, attending the birth and one or two postnatal meetings, with them on call from about 10–14 days before your due date and up to two weeks afterwards. The antenatal appointments are usually about two hours long and are designed to help you get to know each other, cover the essentials of birth preparation and, if this is a second or subsequent birth, run through what happened at your first birth, alleviating any potential worries you might have on the back of it. It is a really good idea to get your partner involved in these appointments. While some women have doulas with them during labour instead of the father, it is just as common that they work alongside the father, involving him in the process at every stage. A good doula will never sideline the father – her role is to make the experience better for everyone.

If you think you might be interested in getting a doula, make sure that you look into it as early as possible. There is a limited number of births a doula can take on in any one year, so they tend to get booked up quite quickly. It is also important that you meet with several people before choosing, to see who you have the best rapport with. Shop around if necessary – while the experience of a doula is important, whether you click with her is even more so. There are now several organisations in the UK that train doulas. Doula UK and Nurturing Birth (see page 269) have quite comprehensive directories of doulas and are a good place to start. Better than Internet shopping is a personal recommendation, however, so ask your yoga for pregnancy, NCT teacher or midwife, and talk to other mothers in the area.

When a dolphin gives birth, an extraordinary thing happens. The mother dolphin is surrounded by an intimate circle of females, all of whom protect her as she labours. Occasionally one of them might intervene, gently nudging the tail of the calf as it emerges from its mother, but generally they simply swim around, forming a barrier between her and the big wide ocean. A little further away, the other female members of the pod form another ring. And then further out still, in a final protective layer, are the males of the pod. In this way, the whole group comes together to nurture the labouring mother, striking a delicate balance between leaving her to birth herself, while providing the necessary protection so that she might do so free from fear and harm.

This is exactly the sort of scenario we need to create if we are to truly relax, let go and labour well. The people by your side in labour have a material impact on how you feel and therefore how you labour. The right birth partner, or support team, can make all the difference. Think of creating your very own dolphin ring to ensure that, whatever happens and wherever you are, you are well supported. For the simple truth is, when a woman's instinctive desire for company and nurture is met, she labours better – usually much, much better.

SUMMARY

- The support you have in labour makes a significant difference to how your labour progresses.
- When you feel secure and emotionally nurtured you will labour more easily and think more positively of your experience.
- One-to-one care has been shown to significantly reduce Caesarean rates, forceps deliveries and the use of medicated pain relief.
- Sometimes this one-to-one care is provided fantastically well by the midwife, but if your care seems more fragmented then it might be useful to consider a doula.
- A doula is a professional birth partner who works alongside the midwife to offer you emotional and physical support leading up to the birth, throughout the entirety of your labour and then postnatally as well. Though she is not medically trained, she has an in-depth understanding of the physiology of birth.
- A huge proportion of fathers also attend the birth of their children, often as sole birth partner, and for most of them it is a wonderful experience to be such an integral part of their child's arrival into the world.
- For some fathers it is, however, an overwhelming prospect and for some mothers an uncomfortable thought that she needs to let go in front of her partner. Have an honest conversation to ensure you are both comfortable with your arrangements for support.

- It is essential that whoever supports you has a good understanding of the birth process and the conditions under which you will labour best. Their role can and might include any or all of the following: advocacy, massage, gentle encouragement, guidance with breathing, reassurance and help in the more active labouring positions.
- Remember that what they do is often less important than their being there.

CHAPTER 4

Pain
The Last Taboo

'In due course, the baby was born. There was no fuss or noise. Everything seemed to have been carried out according to an ordered plan. There was only one slight dissension: I tried to persuade my patient to let me put the mask over her face and give her some chloroform when the head appeared and the dilation of the passages was obvious. She, however, resented the suggestion and firmly but kindly refused to take this help. It was the first time in my short experience that I had ever been refused when offering chloroform. As I was about to leave some time later I asked her why it was that she would not use the mask. She did not answer at once, but looked from the old woman who had been assisting to the window through which was bursting the first light of dawn; and then shyly turned to me and said "It didn't hurt. It wasn't meant to, was it, doctor?"'

Grantly Dick-Read, *Childbirth Without Fear*

Mention the word birth, and the word pain will usually be hot on its heels. While some cultures do not speak of pain in the context of labour, ours is borderline obsessed with it. Since

Queen Victoria first used chloroform for the birth of her son, Leopold, the use of drugs in labour has been both applauded and notorious in equal measure. The feminists hijacked the issue, doctors have grappled with it and *EastEnders'* script-writers make great drama out of it, all the while consolidating in our collective imagination that labour is unbearable and that the only way to deal with the pain is to smother it.

The result is that most pregnant women are more fearful than they need to be about their labours, and fear is a huge impediment – both mental and physical – to a positive birth experience.

In antenatal classes, the approach to pain is usually all or nothing. Most classes deal with the subject by throwing a smorgasbord of pain-relief options at the mother-to-be, assuming that only the truly hardy or crazy will go it alone. Other classes refuse to mention 'pain', as though it is this terrible taboo and to say something would somehow make the whole thing much worse. Neither of these approaches particularly help a mother who is preparing for birth. What you need is an open and head-on look at the issue, one that doesn't give it an exaggerated place in birth, but that doesn't ignore it either.

The Movable Feast

The reassuring thing about the pain of labour is that it is very easily influenced. Far from being some immovable given, a sort of fait accompli, it is hugely determined by our physical comfort and our mental state – and is entirely malleable.

When confronting the pain of labour you can do two things, both of which will help immeasurably:

1 You can change your perception of the pain, which will determine how you cope with it.
2 You can minimise the actual sensations of labour – in both a mental and a physical way.

Where Does the Pain Come From?

The pain of labour is a very normal side-effect of a very normal process. In order to dilate the cervix, the uterus (womb), which is the strongest muscle in the body in terms of mass, needs to contract and to work hard. As with any muscle under the pressure of exertion, this process is not without physical consequence. The thing about labour pain is that it is a product of exertion and not the sometimes inexplicable and therefore frightening pain of illness, and knowing this makes an enormous difference to your capacity to deal with it.

A marathon runner would not deem to say that the running did not involve pain, and mountaineers attest to the sheer physical endurance that they put their bodies through. Hard work, in any context, is not pain free. But what it does not need to be is the defining factor. If pushed, a runner or mountaineer might describe periods of extreme pain, but in their stories it is rarely the emphasis. In the same way, pain can be part and parcel of the birth process but not by any means the whole story.

Understanding the Whole Story

As birth happens largely behind closed doors and our first experience of birth is usually that of our first child, most of what we
know are the soundbites; people's 13-word or less summaries, the
sort that go something like 'long, messy and painful, etc., etc.'
Rarely in their summing up will someone say to you, 'Well the
amazing thing is that contractions are rhythmical, so you have
time in between to recover.' And yet that is exactly how contractions work. Labour is not one long pain. Contractions build up,
then peak, but then they go away. Contrary to what many women
think (and I was one of them) you are not expected to cope with
one long, endless tunnel of agony, but short bursts that you can
breathe through because you know that they will go away. And
believe me this makes a big difference. A huge difference, because
those in-between bits are your lifeline. They give you time to
recover, space to breathe and, the best bit of all, they are when
your body is flooded with a huge cocktail of hormones that
makes you feel not just okay but really quite amazing. In fact,
while the contractions can sometimes be hard to cope with, the
periods in between can be a borderline out-of-body experience.
I bet no one ever told you that!

What's more (and this is the other bit no one tells you), when
the birth is over and done with, and if it hasn't been interfered
with too much, you get an almighty reward (on top of your
baby), which is a high that can last for several days – the result of
all those hormones still coursing through your veins.

NATURE'S OPIATES –
A VERY REASSURING INVENTION

The other part that no one tells you is that we are very well designed for this birth thing. Nature doesn't just throw you into labour without giving you some tools to help. In response to the exertion of labour, the body produces endorphins – sometimes referred to as 'nature's opiates'. This is exactly the same thing that happens to runners, and is the very reason that physical exercise of any sort can become addictive. Endorphins are 500 times stronger than morphine, are said to improve your mood and – get this – have amnesiac qualities, which is why as birth progresses you feel increasingly like you are on another planet or away with the fairies. This is why after a natural birth it is often very difficult to remember the specifics of it. It is also why a lot of women will often say that much to their surprise the earlier part of their labour was more difficult than the later parts, when they were much more out of it and more flooded with endorphins.

It is also the reason why inductions are generally harder to cope with, because they artificially accelerate the labour process, hitting you with contractions that are usually associated with very established labour, before the body has had time to support you with all the necessary hormones and the natural pain relief. And within 20 minutes of having an induction, all your body's natural hormones and pain relief are effectively switched off, which means unless you have further intervention, you will be labouring without all the benefits that nature has created for the birth process.

PAIN HAS A PURPOSE

It is true to say that the pain of labour serves a valuable purpose. And knowing this helps. Pointless pain is infinitely harder to endure than when we know that it is actually helping us. Firstly, feeling your contractions is a cue that labour is beginning, which doesn't sound like a particularly amazing benefit, but, if you think about it, is actually quite useful. Just imagine all the places that babies might be born if we never knew we were in labour!

The discomfort of labour is also often a message for us to move. Women find that they instinctively roll their hips and rotate their pelvis as they have contractions, and in doing so they unwittingly help the descent of their baby through the birth canal. It is not at all uncommon for women in early labour to suddenly want to climb up and down the stairs, and this asymmetrical movement, which rocks the pelvis back and forth, is the ideal movement to swivel the baby into position.

Additionally, the pain is thought to be a positive feedback loop, sending messages to the brain – the pituitary gland in particular – to produce more oxytocin and so keep things moving forward.

PAIN AND SUFFERING ARE NOT
ONE AND THE SAME

As part of my work, I spend an enormous amount of time dealing with the very real and very normal fears that pregnant women have about labour. Pain usually features high on the agenda, but when I dig beneath the banner concerns, it is not so much the pain of labour that women worry about, but the assumption that they will suffer with it. Yet the two are by no means synonymous. Women who wax lyrical about their labour experience will rarely say that it was pain free. And by the same token, I have had many women who have had epidurals come to me afterwards with complaints that in some way they still suffered – anxiety, a lack of emotional support, the feeling that they were alone. The truth is you can suffer without the pain and have pain without the suffering.

In our increasingly cotton-wool world, it is admittedly hard to consider being in pain without also suffering. I confess that I was completely unconvinced prior to the birth of my first child – in fact, the thought of a blood test was enough for me to consider requesting a local anaesthetic. But experience proved me, as it does so many other women, wrong. I was stronger and more capable than I ever thought possible. As one of my earliest students once said to me, 'Giving birth was probably the most difficult and the most testing experience of my life. But it was also, without any doubt, the best.'

In a recent talk, the author and Tibetan Buddhist Sogyal Rinpoche spoke of the absolute necessity for us, as human beings, to develop mental strength. With it, he said, one can have great physical discomfort and still be happy, for the body is ultimately subservient to the mind. His words echo those of the great poet Milton who is famed for saying, 'The mind is its own place. It can make a heaven of hell or a hell of heaven.' The differences between entire cultures of women is not their propensity for pain but their approach to birth and the extent to which birth – with all its attendant discomfort and glory – is considered normal and natural.

Read as many positive birth stories as possible – Ina May Gaskin's *Guide to Childbirth* is full of them, as is Penny Armstrong's

A Wise Birth. Watch good birth DVDs, where women are coping well and whose births are natural. None of this will guarantee you the perfect birth, but it will open your mind to the possibility of one. And in a culture that tends to see birth as a medical condition, it is a very necessary step for the majority of pregnant women.

WHY YOU'LL PROBABLY COPE WITH THE PAIN

- Because it builds up gradually.
- Because until transition (see page 158) the contractions are intermittent so you have time to rest in between them.
- Because the body produces endorphins to help you cope and to make those in-between bits really quite amazing.
- Because it is the pain of endurance not illness.
- Because water, massage, movement and nurture will all reduce the pain you feel.
- Because if you can't cope any more at any point, it is the gloriously modern world and we have pain relief.

The Influence of Expectations

In 1988 a cross-cultural study was done between a group of Dutch and American mothers. The women were all asked about their expectations of pain, and these were then correlated with their eventual birth experience. Not only did the American women expect birth to be considerably more painful, but there was an almost exact match between the women in either group who expected pain and those who used pain relief. In other words, in Holland, where birth is considered more normal, women expected less pain. And across both countries, the women who expected birth to be less painful found that it was. It is almost impossible to determine whether the women who expected less pain actually felt less physically. Measuring what a person actually feels has so far eluded our civilisation. But it would not be beyond the realms of possibility that something in the minds of the more positive women significantly enhanced their capacity to cope.

Supporting this idea is the experience of women with doulas. As we explored in the last chapter, research on continuous care during labour shows that women who are well supported emotionally have much less need for any pain medication – again, who could say that these women feel less pain? Outside of simple comfort measures, a doula's support is largely emotional. Because she is there, a mother is much more likely to be relaxed, so she will not be tensing up and creating unnecessary pain in the body. The mother will also be reassured that what she is feeling is normal and healthy, and so her perception of pain will be altered for the better.

Minimising What You Feel

Assuming that you have now, at least partially, got your head round the pain of labour and where it comes from, as well as what it's for, we can look at ways to minimise what you actually physically feel and suggest some tools that should help you cope.

Pain-free labours are by no means unheard of, but the chances are you are going to feel something, so let's make sure it is manageable for you.

BANISHING THE FEAR

If you are frightened of labour, then you are not the only one. In 2000, 26 per cent of mothers said they felt very worried about pain in childbirth.[22] The truth is, feeling fearful isn't all bad. I think it is useful to feel it at some point during pregnancy because it motivates you to do something about it. Instead of being nonchalant and therefore ultimately unprepared, you can work on your fears and ensure you have dealt with them before labour rather than in the midst of it. It can also prompt really healthy decisions like properly deciding on the right place to give birth, or making the commitment to take on a doula because you know you'll need one. Be assured that just because you are frightened doesn't mean you will have a bad birth experience – so long as you deal with it beforehand. Some of the most frightened mothers end up surprising themselves the most.

Fear during labour is a different matter. It is not useful and, in fact, can be a real impediment to birth. In response to fear the body produces stress hormones (called catecholamines – try saying that quickly 10 times!), which trigger your fight-or-flight response, make your heart beat nineteen to the dozen and your muscles tense up. This can both slow down your labour as well as make your contractions more painful – and obviously we want neither of these things to happen. If, however, you have processed your fears before labour and stay relaxed and breathe well, then your body will produce fewer stress hormones and, instead, feed you with all those lovely endorphins we have been talking about.

IGNORE THE HORROR STORIES

There is a saying in the services industry that a happy customer tells 10 people, whereas an unhappy customer tells 100. It seems to be just the same with birth. Women who have had a bad time seem to shout the loudest, telling everyone they can about it, whereas the ones who have had a good birth whisper it to a select few.

When someone is going to have their appendix out, they are rarely confronted by a scaremonger saying, 'Oooh, well, be careful because I know someone who got septicaemia when they had theirs out,' yet tell people you are pregnant and you don't need to wait long before you are showered with a litany of birth horror stories, all along the lines of 'my sister had a 36-hour nightmare' or 'my friend was in labour for three days and then still ended up having a Caesarean'. Announce that you are thinking of a home birth and you get even more warnings, and even more dire examples of things going wrong.

And TV compounds all of this. A straightforward 12-hour water birth would make very boring viewing. So good births don't get included in the scripts. Instead TV births are full of high drama, with babies born in pub loos, mothers writhing around in apparently inconceivable agony and hapless fathers running around like headless chickens.

So turn off the TV. Definitely do not watch those ghastly daytime birth programmes or the talk-shows that deal with birth in any capacity. They will simply scare you. Decline offers of horror birth stories. And if your protests are ignored and you get to hear one anyway, remember that everyone's experience is different, in all walks of life – just because your friend had a bad experience travelling through Venezuela, doesn't mean you will.

Don't, whatever you do, Google 'birth'. Not under any circumstances. The Internet is awash with good information, no doubt, but most of it is hidden among all the crazy stories, and they will do nothing for your mindset.

Processing Your Fears

In advance of labour there are many ways that you can prepare your mind. First and foremost, it is essential to confront your fears – no matter how seemingly small they might be. Write them down, if necessary, perhaps even ceremonially burn them, as well as speak to your midwife, doula or partner about them. They should be able to reassure you about specific concerns, but quite apart from that, the mere fact of being open and honest about what is bothering you may be enough to allay your worries.

AN EXERCISE IN GETTING RID OF YOUR FEARS

If you are scared of giving birth, then you are by no means alone. Most women express apprehension, while some confess to outright fear. In some ways the fear is healthy, in that it motivates you to do something about it – it is often the impetus for seeking out a class or picking up a book. But lingering fears can get in the way of a good birth, so if you can process them prior to labour, it will only serve you well. A good, and very simple, exercise is to write down what is scaring you on a piece of paper.

You can begin by answering the following questions:

- How do you feel about being pregnant?
- How do you feel about becoming a mother and having a baby?
- Write down, without thinking about it too much, the words you associate with birth.
- Have you ever attended a birth and, if so, what was it like?
- How do you feel when you think about giving birth to this baby?
- What, if anything, excites you about it?
- Is there anything that frightens you?
- If you are in any way fearful, what is it you are frightened of? Be quite specific here.

Once you have written all this down, you can use it in several ways. The first is simple catharsis. Getting something out and down on paper can be hugely helpful. It might sound like hippy clap-trap, but it can also be good to rip your fears into tiny shreds or to ceremonially burn the paper they are written on. A small act, but often a strangely effective one.

You could also use your notes to speak to your midwife about things that might be worrying you. Perhaps it is a long-held fear of hospitals that will then determine where you give birth. Maybe it is a story you heard of someone else's birth and a midwife might be able to reassure you that it is unlikely to happen to you. Perhaps you are fearful that you won't be able to cope and then she can help you to find an antenatal class that might convince you otherwise. And if you have a doula, by all means use what you have written as the basis for a talk with her. Whatever you do with your notes, remember that by being honest and bold you are facing your concerns head on, which is a huge step towards ridding yourself of them.

Sowing Positive Seeds

In the same way that fear can be an impediment to labour and make the whole experience more painful than necessary, positive thinking and harnessing the extraordinary power of the mind can help you have an altogether more positive birth experience.

It is an extraordinary thing to witness a woman who begins to become overwhelmed with her labour literally think or talk herself out of it – and yet it is very real and it absolutely works. I remember spending a significant part of my own labour first time around repeating to myself, 'This pain will not beat me. I am bigger than this.' And a doula client of mine once spent well over an hour reassuring herself with the mantra, 'I am okay, I am okay. I am okay.' Unsurprisingly, she was.

Yoga for pregnancy is also a lovely way to prepare mentally for birth – it works naturally to calm the mind and gives you more control over your thought processes. I cannot tell you how often I have women come to me at 19 weeks pregnant, fearful and tense, only to leave at 41 weeks, head held high and positively relishing the prospect of giving birth. Not all of them have a perfect experience, but that they have conquered their fear undoubtedly helps them through the toughest parts of their labour.

Hypnosis is another wonderful way to soften the mind in advance of labour. The average person thinks of hypnosis as those people on TV shows who are induced to be 'sawn' in half or do something embarrassing in front of a host of laughing strangers. But quackery aside, true hypnosis can be a very powerful tool, sometimes even giving a mother a completely pain-free birth. In her introduction to a talk on 'Natal Hypnotherapy', its founder Maggie Howell described her first experience of hypnosis. A reticent attendee to a study day, she had been encouraged and intrigued by the experience of her husband – a 40-cigarettes-a-day man, who had been hypnotised into giving up. Although she found the subject matter interesting, she remained a self-proclaimed sceptic up until the point where the whole study group, herself included, were hypnotised and then asked to put safety pins through the pinched skins of their arms. Dutifully they did as they were told, and much to her amazement, Maggie felt no pain at all. Understandably surprised, but suitably convinced of the extraordinary power of the mind, she then began to explore the possibility of using hypnosis as a tool for labour pain. And there is no doubt that it is used extremely effectively. Hundreds of women each year sign up to her Natal Hypnotherapy courses as well as to HypnoBirthing courses (which is the Marie Mongon, American equivalent) on offer across the country. The result is a huge proportion of women able to cope amazingly with their birth experiences, all harnessing their minds to good effect. In fact, many midwives will say they can tell that a woman has done hypnosis of some kind during her pregnancy when she appears not to be in labour at all, despite being 6 or 7cm dilated.

Anaesthesia: the Good and the Bad

All well and good you might proclaim. I now understand where the pain comes from and how I might minimise it, and I can even conceive of coping with it, but quite frankly, why should I bother? Anaesthesia is one of the greatest of all human inventions – up there with the wheel, electricity and the proverbial 'sliced bread'. And, what's more, we are the blessed generation, within reach of the 'Rolls-Royce' of anaesthesia, the epidural. Not only do epidurals offer up, in the majority of cases, completely effective pain relief, but babies remain largely unaffected. A mother, once she has been hooked up and administered to, can no longer feel her contractions but she is awake enough to greet her baby, capable of holding and feeding him within moments of birth. Surely, you could quite legitimately ask, isn't it one of those rare 'win–win' situations in life?

The advocates would answer a hearty 'Yes'. I have a friend who lives in Singapore who proclaims, loudly and proudly, that she has given birth three times without ever having felt a contraction. And proud she should be. She has had three positive births and has three healthy boys to show for her endeavours. Birth, with or without drugs, is a feat. It is not for the natural-birth brigade to start dishing out guilt to mothers who decided that they needed an epidural. A well-timed epidural in the right circumstances can mean the difference between a traumatic or a positive birth experience. And after the mother and baby's health, a woman's experience of her birth is hugely important, impacting on her future confidence as a mother and even as a woman. If an epidural truly helps a woman and is something she wants, she should not be denied it, nor should she apologise for it.

The downside is that you don't get something for nothing. The phrase 'no pain, no gain' smacks of an overzealous personal trainer and has the slightly saccharin ring of martyrdom, but it is, rather annoyingly, as true in the context of birth as it is in the world of physical fitness. For there is a genuine and quite compelling upside to being awake to all that birth offers up.

Bonding

That crazy, other worldly, mind-altering high that natural birth produces is a heady synthesis of the cocktail of hormones and endorphins that not only the mother but the baby are flooded with at birth. This naturally helps the early bonding process. After a natural birth, you and your baby are primed to fall in love with one another. When there is intervention, this cocktail is diluted or sometimes even drowned out completely. It doesn't mean mothers and babies who don't have the benefits of this don't bond at all – with time of course they do – but it just means they don't get the head start.

Cascade of Intervention

On a more practical note, choosing to birth without drugs also reduces your exposure to what is known as the 'cascade of intervention'. This is now a well-documented phenomenon and is when one intervention leads to another, and then another. Research has shown that epidurals increase the length of labour, particularly the second stage, as well as increase your chances of having an instrumental delivery or a Caesarean section.[23] If you are knowingly and willingly happy to take on these risks – or if a long or difficult labour has made the decision for you – then by all means take advantage of modern technology. Remember, there are risks to everything we ever undertake. Just make sure that whatever your decisions, they are informed and they are yours.

No Guarantees

Be careful not to assume that smothering the pain of labour will necessarily improve your experience. In fact, studies have shown that more often than not the opposite is the case – for women with uncomplicated labours, even effective forms of pain relief are often not associated with greater levels of satisfaction with the birth experience.

In many ways we are in a blessed position. Birth is potentially safer than it has ever been. We have the luxury of being able to debate all of this because with a mixture of wisdom, medicine and health we have made it so. If after your research you opt for pain relief, do so boldly and without guilt, safe in the knowledge that as an informed decision it is right for you. But remember also that no matter what your choices are on your birth plan (see page 54), you will need to get your head around the idea that your body is going to be doing something tough, and that for a time – even if it is just the time up until you use pain relief – you are likely to feel some sort of discomfort. Rest assured, though, you are more than capable of coping with it, probably much more than you could ever have imagined.

At the very least, it is essential to consider what it means, what it could mean, to be awake and privy to one of the most extraordinary miracles of life. Even the staunchest atheist and most ardent rationalist can still attest to the dizzying heights they are taken to in the process of a truly natural birth. You don't need to be in the least bit religious to recognise that a good birth borders on the sacred. Consider for a moment that the sensations of birth are an aside. Too many women give birth having never entertained the notion that they might enjoy it. And the power of the mind is such that if you think you might, you have taken one giant step closer to it becoming a reality. A wonderful independent midwife by the name of Annie Francis once said to me, 'You will not be sent more pain than you can deal with.' More of us should believe her.

.....

SUMMARY

- The pain of labour is a normal part of a normal process.
- It is the pain of exertion not of illness.
- Fear – or anything else that creates tension in the body – increases unnecessarily the pain of labour.
- The more you can relax and breathe well, the less pain you will feel.
- The quality of support you get in labour has a direct impact on the pain you will feel. In many cases, a good birth partner is as good as any drug.
- Pain relief is widely available and for many women means the difference between a good and a bad birth experience, but remember that your chances of further intervention are significantly increased if you have an epidural.
- Your body is cleverly designed to produce its own natural pain relief, which means that many women cope far better than they might ever have imagined.
- The upside to a natural birth is the extraordinary flood of endorphins and oxytocin that you get, leaving you on the sort of high marathon runners and mountain climbers get.

CHAPTER 5

Water Birth
Riding the Waves

'Nothing in the world is as soft and yielding as water, and yet in dissolving the hard and inflexible, nothing can surpass it.'
Lao Tzu, *Tao Te Ching*

People have long recognised the therapeutic properties of water. All over the world hot springs are visited for rejuvenation, and steam rooms and spas are renowned for their capacity to calm and heal. Good garden design always incorporates water in some form or another, be it a cooling pond or a trickling stream, and for many people the world over, the perfect antidote to physical exertion or sore muscles is a long soak in a hot bath or a revitalising swim in the ocean. In fact, so widespread is the use of water across cultures that it is perhaps surprising that birthing mothers have been so late to the game.

In some cultures this love of water has always found its way into the birth arena – there are stories of Japanese women in fishing villages who naturally birth by the sea, and of Finnish women labouring in steaming saunas. In parts of Africa, the steam from hot rocks is used specifically to soften the perineum, while Guatemalan midwives speak of using hot baths and massage as a way of commonly alleviating discomfort in labour. In the West, however, using water as an aid to birth is still relatively novel. The particular geography of a country must play its part – it should come as no surprise that water is far from the mind of a labouring woman in Mongolia, where the first ever water birth occurred as late as 2007! Being an island, the UK has no such excuse, though our particular brand of rainy and cold climate makes waterways entirely unenticing for birth. Hence the need for the rather wonderful invention of the birthing pool, brought as an idea to our shores in the 1980s and increasingly in use ever since.

The benefits of using water during labour have now been well documented: significantly shorter labours, a much reduced need for pain relief, a much happier experience for the mother and a gentle entry into the world for the baby. In fact, this list is not exhaustive. Staying in the water for the second stage has also been shown to reduce the incidence of tearing.[24] With so many benefits, the only surprise should be that water is not more commonly used. A small postal survey done between 1994 and 1996 suggested only 1 per cent of births were water births at the time.[25] Even if this figure is now wildly out, it still means that the vast majority of women in the UK are not even considering it. Yet they should be. If you are after a normal, healthy and natural birth, water should be, at the bare minimum, a consideration.

The Benefits of Water for Labour

1) SHORTER LABOURS

The biggest major study on the use of water during labour concluded that water *reduces the length of labour by two hours on average*.[26] When you understand the physiology of natural birth, it makes perfect sense. In water you will be calmer, more physically and mentally relaxed, less exposed and subject to much less sensorial stimulation. This all means that your front brain (see page 13) is much more likely to stay switched off, and you are much less likely to produce any of the hormone adrenaline, which specifically hinders the first stage of labour (see page 140). In fact, the soothing impact of water is so acute for some women that even the sound of water has been known to have sped up their labours. In my work as a doula I have often seen a woman's face take on an almost beatific air when she sinks down into the warm water for the first time. What's more, a well-timed entry into the water pool can speed up labour just when things are getting tough, making what had become unmanageable manageable once again.

As one mother said to me, 'It didn't take all the sensations away, but it took the edge off it all. Once I was in the water I could cope again.'

And another mother was even more adamant: 'I couldn't believe the effect of the water. There I was thinking I simply couldn't go on, and then I got into the water and it was like a different labour. Suddenly I was coasting along again, just breathing through contractions and coping as though the clocks had been turned back.'

The timing of water use is, in fact, crucial, and it is something I think carers very often get wrong. The idea is not to loll around in a bath for hours on end. Often after having sped things up in the first two hours, water can actually begin to slow things down, so you don't want to be in there forever.[27] It is best to wait until absolutely necessary, so that you are as far along in your labour as possible and have used up all your own resources first. There is, after all, no point in going quickly from 4 to 6 cm dilated when there is still so much more to go. So hold on until you feel you really need to be in the water and then you will fully maximise the benefits. In fact, many childbirth educators say that it's when you might want to shout for an epidural that it is the perfect time to get into the water. I would add that there will just come a time when you know you need something more.

2) LESS NEED FOR PAIN RELIEF

To say that water is a viable alternative to other forms of pain relief is no exaggeration. *Women who use water are much less likely to ask for any other pain relief.* One study looked at a group of first-time mothers and found that only 24 per cent of those who laboured in water needed pain-relieving drugs as compared to 50 per cent of those who did not use water. Other studies back this finding, with some showing that 100 per cent of the mothers who used water needed no other form of pain relief. So convincing is the use of water, that it is now argued that it is the second most effective form of pain relief after epidurals and is often dubbed the 'aquadural'. It makes simple common sense. Where is the best place to be if you have done something back-breaking (like digging in the garden) or have just run what felt like a marathon? A warm bath. There is nothing better for muscular discomfort. In fact, warmth alone is so useful that I always advise packing a hot-water bottle in your birth bag, or having one on hand at home, to use on your lower back during the early stages of labour. A strategically placed hot-water bottle, nestled into the lower back and held in place by a willing birth partner, can be of huge comfort in the earlier stages when it's too early to jump in the bath. Another good way to use water before the full swim is by having a warm and preferably high-pressure shower during early labour. If we think of pain as a competition between small nerve fibres, which carry labour pain, and large nerve fibres (the skin), which will be stimulated by water and warmth, then we can see why water cascading on to your skin will help to reduce any pain and discomfort. If you are in the shower, try to direct the spray at the base of your spine and make sure that you have something to hold on to, or are well supported.

Rest assured that the water, once you get in it, will be warm. The pool needs to be kept just slightly cooler than body temperature. A big concern voiced by mothers I teach is that they might feel cold, or that the water might run lukewarm (I can think of few things I like less than a not quite hot enough bath!), but midwives know that it is essential to keep it between 34 and 36°C for labour and a little warmer (between 37 and 37.5°C) for the delivery itself. The midwife will keep topping it up if necessary. If you are at home, make sure the boiler stays on and that you have access to warm water all the time.

3) HELPS YOU TO STAY ACTIVE IN LABOUR

Having a truly active birth is made infinitely easier in water. One of the downsides of an active birth is that it requires significant strength and stamina on your part. This is made much easier by being in water – its natural buoyancy means you can labour upright for longer without running out of puff and without needing as much physical support from those around you. Adopting those lovely primal positions and changing from one to another – which is usually no mean feat at 40+ weeks pregnant – is also much easier in water, so positions that on land might be out of bounds can be added to your repertoire. This is good as it gives you more ways to shift your baby through the birth canal and a much greater sense of control over your own body.

In fact, being in control of your own experience is hugely enhanced in water, it seems. One woman came back to class to tell her birth story and said that while in labour she had discovered an unexpected benefit to water. When a clock-watching doctor came into her room and asked if she could get out of the pool to be internally examined, she simply pushed off to the other side of the pool, with an almighty shake of the head. 'I had specified that I didn't want any internal examinations,' she said, 'and because I was in the water he couldn't chase me!'

Having said that, the essential monitoring that needs to be done by a midwife throughout labour is not hindered by you being in water. Between contractions your baby's heartbeat will be listened to with a waterproof sonic aid. These are the same as the Dopplers that midwives use at antenatal check-ups when they listen for your baby's heartbeat – the only difference being that they can go under water. If a baby is to be born in the water and the midwife wants to monitor progress, then she will use a mirror (and sometimes a torch, too), angling it to see the baby's head as it emerges.

4) ENHANCES YOUR SENSE OF PRIVACY

Another benefit to water is that your privacy is dramatically increased once you get in. If you imagine the contrasting experience (and levels of potential embarrassment) between someone walking in on you in the bathroom when you are standing fully naked and upright, as compared to accidentally trespassing while you are fully submerged in the bath, water begins to make sense for those who might find the whole nakedness thing an issue during labour. A lot of women are completely comfortable with the idea of taking their clothes off for birth and you might be one of them, but many others express an acute discomfort with

WAYS TO USE WATER
- Drink it through a bendy straw.
- Shower in it in the early stages.
- Use it in a hot-water bottle nestled into your back.
- Bath in it from when you are 5 or 6 cm dilated.
- Spray it on your face if you get hot.
- Dip your feet in it to soothe and distract you.
- Use it to make a hot or cold flannel to put across your brow or at the nape of your neck.

it. If you are in the latter camp, firstly don't feel at all strange – it's quite normal to feel this way – and then seriously consider labouring in water. Though you need to take your clothes off to get in there, once you are in, the water can provide a lovely aquatic den that protects your sense of modesty without hindering your ability to move or to birth your baby.

Water and the Second Stage

Whether you stay in the water during the second stage depends partly on hospital policy – in some places they are happier if you get out – and partly on how you feel. Some women are so happy in the water that it would take a crane to remove them (that was me!), while others feel a sudden urge to feel gravity and the earth beneath them to birth their baby.

If you decide to stay in, there are benefits to doing so: a reduced risk of tearing, a reduced sensation when your baby's head crowns, and then a gentle entry into the world for your baby.

If you do remain in the water for the birth, then just like on dry land, it is likely that the baby's head is born first after which there will be a pause before the next contraction, when the shoulders will be born. Do not worry at this stage that your baby's head is under water, as he will not be breathing conventionally and will still be fed oxygen through the placenta. In fact, the reason it is possible for babies to be born under water safely is because of something called the 'dive reflex'. The breathing reflex of a baby is stimulated after birth, when sensory chemoreceptors located around the nose and mouth first come into contact with air. Until this point, the placenta is still responsible for providing the baby with oxygen, as it did in the womb when the baby was swallowing amniotic fluid. When the baby is born into warm water during a water birth, this stimulation does not occur until the baby's face is brought to the surface of the water. Until this time the larynx is closed and any water that enters the baby's nose or mouth is simply swallowed rather than inhaled. The only time this 'dive reflex' might be overridden is if a baby were in distress, which is why women are not advised to use water if there is evidence that the baby has passed meconium (see page 225) or if the labour is not progressing normally. In all other circumstances, water has so far been found to be safe.

Once the baby's shoulders and body have been born, which is usually one contraction after the head is born, then the baby can gently be brought to the surface either by yourself or your midwife. It is important to keep the baby's little body submerged so that he stays warm and to make sure the room is sufficiently warm before you leave the pool. As the birth has not finished (the placenta still needs to be born), it is important to keep the room dark and quiet and to maintain respect for the mother's privacy. As in a land birth, you will be encouraged to allow the baby to suckle to stimulate the birth of the placenta. Sometimes it is advisable to leave the water for the third stage of labour; it is best to seek the advice of your midwife.

For those who choose to get out of the water for the birth itself, the mild change in temperature from the water to the air is often enough to initiate the surge of adrenaline that occurs naturally during transition (the cold causes the body to produce adrenaline) and leads to babies often being born very quickly after a woman leaves the pool.

Whatever happens, when considering labouring in water, it is essential to remain open-minded, especially about whether to actually give birth in the water. Check out your hospital's policy and speak to your midwife about the possibility of remaining in the water for the second stage. Remember, also, that you don't know how you are going to feel on the day – your instincts, as well as the midwife's advice, will help you to make the right decision.

With so many documented benefits, it should not be surprising that women who labour in water speak highly of their birth experience. The odd mother is not enamoured. I have one particular friend who called me up to speak with great glee about her second birth, but with the postscript that she couldn't understand all my fuss about water. 'I felt no different,' she proclaimed, almost crossly, 'except that I was wet!' She, however, is the exception rather than the rule. The vast majority of women who labour in water say they would do so again. Usually they are almost evangelical about it.

The push for water as a choice has predominantly come from women themselves, who through the grapevine have heard of its benefits and want to have something available to them that is non-invasive. In response, hospitals and birthing centres across the country now have birth pools and, increasingly, midwives are well versed in the art of water birth. Countless places hire out water pools for those choosing to birth at home, and many a woman opts for a home birth to ensure she has access to a pool. I have included a couple of good links and addresses should you be interested in a water birth and need a pool (see page 269).

SUMMARY

- Water has been used for centuries for its therapeutic properties.
- More recently women have been using water for labour and birth.
- It is so effective as a form of pain relief that it has been dubbed 'the alternative epidural'.
- Water reduces the length of labour, improves the experience for the labouring mother and enhances her ability to have an active birth.
- Some mothers choose to give birth, as well as labour, in water, which reduces the incidence of tearing and is a gentle entry into the world for the baby.
- Studies so far have shown that water birth is a safe alternative to giving birth on dry land.

CHAPTER 6

Optimal Foetal Position
Not One for the Feminists …

'Nature goes to great lengths to help babies make the best choice!'
Jean Sutton, *Let Birth be Born Again*

As the baby's journey through the birth canal is a series of twists and turns – as opposed to a simple case of passing through a tunnel – the position the baby starts in and how she negotiates the move through the inlet and outlet of the pelvis is relevant to how labour progresses. In fact, many midwives will say it is not size but position that is everything when it comes to birth. This is why from about 32 weeks a midwife will often palpate (manually feel for) the baby's position.

The Anatomy of the Pelvis

The reason for the baby having to make this rather bendy journey is that the pelvis is not the same diameter at the top and the bottom. The inlet, or opening, of the pelvis is wider from side to side, so well-positioned babies will begin the birth journey with the widest diameter of their heads – front to back – aligned with this. The outlet, or exit, of the pelvis is widest from front to back, which is why a baby will in most cases spiral around to line the back of the head up with the pubic arch.

As the baby needs to twist and turn to make best possible use of the available space, the start position is key. Parallel parking a car is a good analogy. If we start to park and try to go nose in first, even seemingly large spaces seem non-negotiable. Pull up ahead of the space and back in, and even the tightest spot becomes a possibility. The size of the car matters less than the position it starts in. Another good example of position making all the difference is if you are trying to put on or take off a turtle-neck jumper. Put it over your brow, the wide part of the head, and getting your jumper on is a hideous process that drags on your ears and in all likelihood gets stuck halfway. Tuck your chin in and try to pull the jumper over the back of your head, and suddenly the very same process is as easy as pie. (Unsurprisingly, and for the very same reason, babies tend to instinctively tuck their chins in and present this smaller part of their head first.) The point is, since the advent of modern nutrition and well-fed mothers, with well-formed pelvises, the issue of being born – if there is one – is rarely the available space but more how the baby manoeuvres through it.

All well and good you might say, but how do you have any control over the way in which your baby negotiates the pelvic inlet? You can hardly get in there with her and go along for the ride!

As we talked about in chapter two, being active in labour can be of huge help to this spiralling action of the baby (see page 36);

very often a woman's instinct to circle her hips or to climb the stairs is an unknowing attempt to help the journey. But just as important as understanding the benefits of an active labour is knowing that the position the baby begins from is relevant. Before we look at the detail, however, just a few words of caution. Midwives, and therefore also the women they are looking after, can get obsessed with a baby's position. While in some cases this is justified (ascertaining if a baby is breech, for example), in many cases it simply causes undue worry on the part of the mother. Although babies begin to settle into position from as early as 32 weeks, they still have plenty of time to move before labour begins and especially so in a second or subsequent pregnancy. It might be interesting to work out which poke is a foot and which flutter a hand, but it should not be a cause for concern if you are still weeks away from your due date.

The second thing to remember is that while there are some things that mothers can do to help their babies into the perfect position – and we will discuss all of these in a moment – there are occasionally babies who will not budge no matter what happens or who, for no apparent reason, will change position at the last minute. You can influence the positioning of your baby to a degree, but fixating on it is likely to cause you undue stress. Rest assured, with some vigilance on your part, most babies get themselves into a good position and the vast majority stay there. So what are the different positions a baby can be in, and what difference do they make?

Cephalic versus Breech

The first major distinction is cephalic (head down) versus breech (bottom down). The only alternative to these two is what is known as a transverse lie, where the baby is lying side to side or across the mother's belly. This is very rare but it is also an unequivocal reason for a Caesarean section unless the baby can be turned.

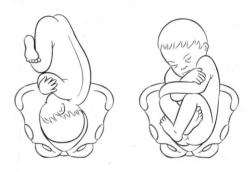

If your baby is diagnosed as breech at about 32 weeks, then the chances are she will turn of her own accord – only 3 per cent of babies are breech at term, yet 25 per cent are diagnosed as breech at 32 weeks. If yours still hasn't moved by around 36 weeks, then you might want to consider some of your options for turning the baby.

WAYS TO TURN A BREECH BABY

There are a number of exercises you can try to turn a breech baby; the following are the three most common:

Knee–chest position
This is the best position to use to try to turn your baby. Get on to all fours, and check that your knees are directly beneath your

hips and your hands are beneath your shoulders. This position in itself is good for encouraging a baby into the optimal foetal position, and I am a big advocate of women regularly using it in the latter stages of their pregnancy for periods during the day. It is an integral part of any yoga class I teach.

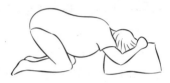

From all fours, try to bring your chest to the floor, leaving your hips and bottom sticking up in the air. Turn your head to one side so that you can get your cheek to the floor, and bend your elbows so that you can bring your arms down. Relax your shoulders, breathe gently and stay in this position for as long as feels comfortable, working up to about 20-minute stints, three times a day. To alleviate boredom, play some music (or a birth or hypnotherapy CD) or try to angle yourself so that you can watch TV. Make sure you tell your partner what you are doing, and trying to achieve, in case he thinks you have simply lost your mind in a fit of pregnancy-related lunacy! An initial report into the benefits of this method was very encouraging, though subsequent studies have been less so. As it can't hurt, I suggest giving it a try.

Acupuncture
Another method that has been used to turn babies for many years is acupuncture, with very good results. The treatment for breech babies involves using a moxa (a type of herb) stick, which looks like a cigar. It is burnt to warm the acupuncture point at the side

of the little toe on the right foot. The treatment is repeated on alternate days until the baby has turned. It is obviously important to seek out a professional acupuncturist for this treatment, though he or she will often send you home with moxa sticks of your own. You can also stimulate the relevant acupuncture point by massaging the outer part of the little toe several times a day for up to three minutes, but do not do this if you are undergoing a specific acupuncture treatment. It might sound a rather strange process, especially to those who have not used acupuncture before, but the success rate with this form of treatment is very good, with informal studies showing that up to 75 per cent of babies turn. It is best to undertake it at around 33 or 34 weeks of pregnancy when the baby still has ample room to turn around.

External Cephalic Version

The most common way that breech babies are turned is through a process called External Cephalic Version (ECV) which is a manual turning of a baby from breech (bottom down) to cephalic (head down). It is usually undertaken at 36 weeks for first babies and 37 weeks for second and subsequent babies after a scan has ascertained that the baby is indeed breech. This confirmation is necessary, and arguably increasingly so. Midwives will not like me for saying this, but in my experience, wrong diagnoses of breech babies are becoming more and more frequent. As we become increasingly reliant on scans for diagnosing positions of babies, palpating (the manual means of diagnosis) is becoming something of a lost art. Some midwives are still very adept, but more and more seem to confuse bottoms and heads. And by all accounts it is very easy to do. Baby's bottoms are tiny and relatively fat free in the womb, so confusing a bony bottom and a bony head is not difficult.

The scan is also to ascertain if something unusual is causing the baby to be breech. Most babies are breech for no particular reason at all, but occasionally it is due to an excess of amniotic fluid, a baby being small for its age or because of a low-lying placenta that is getting in the way. Obviously scans can rule these causes out and if all looks normal, then the procedure can begin. In some hospitals a drug is used to relax the uterine walls, and then an obstetrician will manually manipulate and massage the abdomen to guide the baby through a forward somersault. Some women claim the procedure can be uncomfortable, even painful at times, but the 60 per cent success rate is enough to convince most that it is worth a try. The baby's heartbeat is monitored throughout, and after the procedure the vast majority of babies that are turned don't turn back.

If your baby is persistently breech then it is possible to opt for a vaginal birth regardless, depending on hospital policy and the experience and inclination of your midwife or obstetrician. It is well worth discussing your options with your caregivers, based on your own preferences. Alternatively, a caesarean section will be scheduled some time after week 37.

Anterior versus Posterior

Your baby will be lying in an anterior or posterior position. Anterior is when the baby is lying head down, with her spine to the mother's belly. On your notes the midwife might well break down the distinction further, detailing whether the baby is lying to the left (LOA in your notes) or the right (ROA) of your spine. While either of these positions is good at the beginning of labour, it is believed that LOA is the optimum as the baby is slightly more likely to turn posterior from the right side. A posterior position is when the baby is lying head down, but with her spine to the mother's spine – which is why it is sometimes called the 'back-to-back' position. The distinction is also often made between LOP (left) and ROP (right).

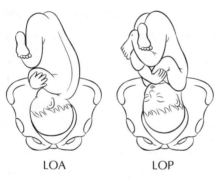

LOA   LOP

For the pregnant mother, the distinction between an anterior or posterior position is probably the more important one to focus on, mainly because it is one that we can influence – for better or for worse – during our pregnancy.

POSTERIOR BIRTHS: ON THE UP

There is an argument to suggest that the whole feminist movement has been good for our pay packets but not so good for our births. When Jean Sutton, a no-nonsense New Zealand midwife at the forefront of discussions regarding positioning of babies, first began working as a district nurse some 60 years ago, she claimed that posterior-positioned babies were as rare as hens' teeth. In her first year of work aged just 17 she presided over 200-odd births, only one of which needed 'rescue' by forceps. Now she believes that in as many as half of all the births she attends, babies are in a posterior position and that their mothers have much harder labours because of it. Other studies suggest a more modest figure of about 30 per cent, but whoever you believe, the number is high. And higher, many people argue, than it needs to be.

The problem is, posterior births are much more difficult. Firstly, they tend to be a lot slower. From an anterior (the ideal) position, contractions push the crown of the baby's head down on to the cervix, putting pressure on the cervix to open. This pressure also sends strong signals to the mother's brain to produce more of that fantastic cocktail of hormones, which keeps labour going. From the posterior position, the baby's head can't help with cervical dilation because it is the broader, flatter, middle part of the baby's head that is lying against the cervix, so the pressure is not as even or as strong. This is why persistently irregular or unusually short contractions can sometimes be a sign of a posterior baby.

The likelihood of intervention is much highter in slower births, leading to the possibility of the dreaded 'cascade of intervention' (see page 98).

Posterior births also tend to be much more painful for the mother. From the optimal (anterior) position a baby needs to simply slip into the pelvis, whereas from a posterior position the baby has to do a lot of turning before she can effectively begin that spiralling descent. As the baby turns, her head passes across the sacrum, an area very rich in nerve endings, which is why women with posterior labours often complain of an experience that is dominated by sensations – often really unbearable ones – in the lower back.

So why this apparent huge increase in the number of posterior births? It is believed that it has an enormous amount to do with how we spend our time. When we hunted and gathered for food, which in the whole scheme of things really wasn't that long ago, women were constantly bent forward – picking berries, hunched over fires or bent over rudimentary brooms. In tribal cultures, where life is lived at a subsistence level, women still spend much of their life leaning forward, tending crops and working physically, very often with a baby strapped to their back. Even our more immediate forebears, our grandmothers and great-grandmothers, will have spent a disproportionate amount of time leant over a wash tub or a sink or down on their knees scrubbing floors and tending vegetables.

The modern mother, on the other hand, tends to take transport rather than walk, has the luxury of white goods to wash her clothes and dishes, and very often has the same sedentary job as her male counterparts. And since the advent of TV, her leisure time is increasingly spent slumped on the sofa.

Whereas before all the bending forward encouraged a baby to rotate around into the optimal foetal position, now many of our babies swivel the other way, to where they can lie comfortably. The truth is we might well have burnt our bras and freed ourselves from the drudgery of the traditional woman, but in doing so there is a good chance that some of us have also blockaded our births.

There is, I assure you, no need to give up the vote. I am not in any way, God forbid, arguing for getting women back into their pre-60s' barefoot, pregnant and in the kitchen state. But the truth is, anecdotal evidence suggests the more active your lifestyle, the less likely you are to have a posterior baby.

Second and subsequent births are less likely to be posterior. It is possible that there is simply more room for babies to manoeuvre second and third time round, and they are more likely to engage later in the pregnancy. But it could also be the case that as the second-, third- or fourth-time mother is running around after a small child (or lots of small children), she is in all likelihood more active and spending much more of her time bent forward in the traditional 'womanly' way!

Making the Baby Comfortable

Remember, while babies are cocooned in amniotic fluid, they will tend to move to where it is comfortable. So on a day-to-day basis, try to be aware of where you are making it comfortable for the baby to go. A good way to think of it is to imagine that the baby is lying happily in a hammock. You can either 'make' a hammock of your belly, with lots of leaning forward positions, or a hammock of your spine or back, with lots of lying back positions. If you think in terms of the first option, making your belly that very comfortable hammock, then these are the positions you should be tending towards.

TRANSPORT

Cars are a fairly dreaded enemy with regard to the position of your baby. The seats in cars are like buckets, and tend to thrust the pelvis back and the shoulders forward. If you can reduce the amount of time you spend in the car, then by all means do so, but for some pregnant women this is not an option. If you have to drive, have a cushion wedged into the base of the seat. If it is there permanently, you won't risk forgetting it, and it will stop the seat from being quite so bucket-like and tilting your pelvis backwards. It will also probably make you look like a bit of a granny at the wheel, all up close and peering, but some things, like reducing your labour by 12 hours, are worth it. If your preferred mode of transport is a train, then take a cushion with you to place beneath your pelvis or in the small of your back.

WORKING

At your desk consider sitting on a birth ball instead of a chair – these are absolutely fabulous for positioning the baby as it is nigh on impossible to slump back on them. If it isn't high enough to use at a desk then you can put a cushion on top of it. The main things to be conscious of when using a ball are that your knees are lower than your pelvis and that your feet can be flat on the floor. Alternatively, you can use one of those chairs designed for bad backs that you kneel on, as they will tilt your pelvis forward in the same way. If neither of those is an option, then sit on the edge of a rolled-up towel and place a small cushion in the small of your back to try to get the same effect. If you are at home, you can use the same ideas, propping yourself up with cushions on the sofa or, better still, sitting on the floor with your back supported by the base of the sofa.

SLEEPING

Try to sleep on your left-hand side as much as possible, or for afternoon naps you could even create a nest of cushions to allow you to sleep face down. It is not a problem to sleep face down during pregnancy as long as your belly is well supported.

YOGA

Try to get yourself to yoga for pregnancy classes because they have been stripped of all positions that require lying on your back, and by its very nature yoga improves your posture helping to rotate the baby. Regular swimming is also really good, as it has you in a horizontal position, making the perfect hammock of your belly. There are some who argue that breaststroke legs are good for positioning a baby, but any pelvic pain is going to be exacerbated by the breaststroke kick, so I would always err on the side of caution and kick your legs front-crawl style. Chiropractors complain incessantly about breaststroke, pregnant or not, because of the way in which it unnaturally curves the spine – who would have thought simple swimming could be such a minefield?

If by week 37 your baby is not in the optimal position, then try not to worry – there are things you can still try. For the most part, try to spend time in inverted, forward-leaning postures. The idea behind this is to be:

1 Upside down, to stop the baby from engaging until she gets into a good position.
2 Forward leaning, to encourage that very position.

When you do anything to try to move the baby, wait until she is awake – by this stage you should be able to determine periods of movement and periods of rest. A baby that is awake is going to be much more responsive than one that is sleeping – which sounds really obvious but you'd be surprised how many people don't think of it! It is also a good idea to do the positions whenever you feel Braxton Hicks as these mild 'practice' contractions will facilitate any rotation.

The process of the baby turning could well be a little bit uncomfortable. Not horribly so, but enough that without thinking you might wriggle around or lean back, which will hinder the baby's ability to move. Just breathe nice and deeply and allow the baby to turn. It might sound crazy, but visualising the baby actually making the move can also be hugely helpful. Have a warm bath, give your belly a gentle massage and encourage the baby to roll over.

There is a host of positions that you can use – handstands in the pool was one that I read about, but have yet to find someone who has actually done it! The yoga position 'downward dog' is also a good one as is the knee–chest position described on page 115.

If all of this doesn't work, and you have a baby that is persistently posterior, then you might need to adjust your expectations of birth. A natural birth – if that is something you were hoping for – is by no means unattainable. I know plenty of women who have had posterior births in much the same way they intended, but that simply took a lot longer. But recognise, also, that it might prove a more difficult experience than you had anticipated, and be open-minded to possibility and change throughout your labour. Posterior births are possible without pain relief, but do not in any way think you have 'failed' if you opt for an epidural or some other relief – it might be the difference between a positive and negative birth experience, and remember that there are no medals dished out for birth bravery. Do what is right for you.

Make sure that you have all the support you can get and really consider having more than one birth partner so that you can be assured of complete continuity of care. If your labour is long, you will want support throughout. Ask your partner (or partners) for a good, firm lower-back massage, or simply strong pressure on the sacrum. A wonderful yoga teacher of mine, who looked after her sister through labour, used the thin ends of two wooden spoons to apply specific pressure on the sacrum the entire way through her sister's 18-hour labour. I have also heard of doulas using tennis balls to spare their hands from cramping up, pressing them and rolling them over the base of the mother's sacrum and giving her wonderful relief for the period that the baby is turning. They sound like simple tools and simple techniques, but they shouldn't be underestimated.

Try to get the baby to turn in early labour. Spend up to 45 minutes in the knee–chest position (see page 115). Avoid having your membranes ruptured if at all possible. This is because to turn from posterior to anterior, a baby needs to rotate a full 180 degrees (usually it's just 90) – intact waters provide a cushion to turn on and so will help the process.

Most of all try not to worry too much. It is perfectly possible, and not at all uncommon, that a baby who has been persistently posterior for weeks turns at the last minute and gets into the best possible position for the onset of labour. Believe that your baby will do just that and it just might happen.

SUMMARY

- Your baby's position is a key determinant of how your labour will unfold.
- We have, to a degree, the ability to influence this position.
- The best possible position for a baby is lying on the left-hand side, with the spine to your belly.
- More and more babies are posterior and it is believed that our sedentary lives are in part to blame.
- It is important throughout pregnancy to use forward-leaning postures as much as possible to help nudge the baby into the optimal position.
- Whenever possible, sit with a small cushion or rolled-up towel beneath your pelvis.
- Try as much as possible to sleep on your left-hand side.
- If your baby is not in the correct position approaching birth, try not to fret – many babies move around at the last minute, and there are exercises you can do to help them.
- If your baby is persistently posterior, then be prepared for a longer labour and make plans accordingly. Pressure on the sacrum can be hugely helpful throughout the first stage of a posterior labour. You might also want to consider an epidural if your baby is persistently posterior.

PART 2
The Birth

CHAPTER 7

The Labyrinth vs the Maze
How Labour Unfolds

'Birth – as experienced by the mother – is the Mount Everest of physical functions. Unless we have seen it before, we can barely imagine that something so relatively huge can come out of a place that looks so small. And yet, it happens every day.'
Ina May Gaskin, *Ina May's Guide to Childbirth*

There is a subtle yet fundamental difference between a maze and a labyrinth. A maze is specifically designed to get you lost, misleading you with dead-ends and choices that lead to them. You very often have to retrace your footsteps and there is always the danger that you might, if you are hopelessly unlucky or spatially unaware, never find your way out. A labyrinth is similar in that it winds and bends and twists, but if you stay the course and simply follow the path, you will always get to the end. It might feel at times as though you will never get there, or even at times as though you are getting further from your goal, but as long as you keep going you will get there in the end.

Modern birth is often depicted as a maze. Women are made to believe that they can't do it without a lot of help and serious intervention. It is depicted as something complex, or even worse, something that we are – as a species – not very good at. But this is a misrepresentation. Birth is actually like a labyrinth, and to think of it as such can be a really useful psychological tool. It won't necessarily always be easy, and there might be times when you feel that you are lost or that you cannot go on, but it is a journey, with a beginning, a middle and an end, and every step you take is one closer to the ultimate prize – your baby.

First and foremost, we need to trust in the process, to trust what our bodies are doing and that our instincts know what to do. As Ina May Gaskin says, birth is the Mount Everest of physical functions yet it is happening all the time.[28] There are around 300 babies born worldwide every minute. We have been reproducing as a species for millions of years. Birth is something that, contrary to popular belief, we are actually quite good at. And when giving birth in the West, we have the added bonus that if natures proves unruly – which for a small minority it might – then we have the medical back-up and the technology to help. Birth has never been safer.

It cannot be overemphasised that a positive mental state from the outset does wonders for your ability to cope with birth. We have been so horribly bombarded with slogans from the self-help industry, that there is a tendency to throw the baby out with the bath water, and thereby completely disregard the extraordinary capacity of our mind to determine our experience. Yet we are what we think. The mind and body are inextricably linked, and never more so than during a natural birth.

PRE-LABOUR

'A woman awaits the event of birth, and prepares for it for 10 lunar months. Nevertheless, it always comes unexpectedly.'
Tatyama Sargunas, Russian Midwife

The Tyranny of the Due Date

No matter how much you advise a woman otherwise, she will in all likelihood get fixated on her due date. Tell her that the average woman is five days late, or that in France gestation is considered 41 weeks (both true) and still she will count down the days, almost like a child waiting for Christmas, and is very likely to feel impatient and overdue by the time she gets there. Only the seriously carefree are more whimsical about it. And, to be fair, it is entirely understandable. One of the first things we do when we find out we are pregnant is calculate our due date. And then the midwife does it again. And then the scan confirms or moves it. And then we write it in our diary, we tell everyone who asks, we even work out what star sign it makes our unborn baby.

And then 40 weeks on, when we are cumbersome and laden, barely able to sleep and incapable of tying our own shoelaces, we are borderline desperate for that baby to be born, and every extra day feels like an eternity.

So what I am going to say now is in all likelihood going to fall on deaf ears, but I'll say it anyway. Be patient.

....

Fruit ripens in its own time. Babies bake in theirs. An unripe avocado might be nudged along by being put in a brown paper bag with a banana, but it will still ripen when it is good and ready. Rest assured, you won't stay pregnant forever.

If you are trying hard to be patient but are desperate to do something (and perhaps ward off induction at the same time), then there are some things – like the brown paper bag for avocados – that might help nudge things in the right direction. The science behind a lot of these methods is fairly indifferent, and a lot are simple old wives' tales, but as I always say to the women I teach, if it can't hurt where's the harm in trying. Science has proved old wives' tales true in the past. And if the impact is nothing more than psychological – the good old placebo effect – then you'll take that I am sure.

What to Do When you Are Overdue
GO WALKING

It might just be my imagination, but there always seem to be more overdue babies in the winter. And if it is true, this little theory of mine, then I suspect it has to do with the fact that we are generally more sedentary in the winter. For there is no doubt that walking is one of the best ways to get labour going. It won't ripen a stubborn cervix, but it will help get the baby into a good position and harness gravity to increase the pressure of the baby's head on the cervix, both of which need to happen to kick-start labour. So a daily, long(ish) walk is a good place to start in the weeks and days leading up to your due date and beyond.

Just make sure that when you are only days away from your due date, or overdue, you walk with someone or don't stray too far from home, and you have your mobile phone with you. I have known of at least one mother whose labour kicked off halfway around a long circular walk!

DRINK RASPBERRY LEAF TEA

From 36 weeks of pregnancy it is advisable to drink several cups of raspberry leaf tea a day. This helps tone the uterus, which helps to make your contractions more effective and your labour more steady. The tea works better if it has time to build up, so drinking it several weeks in advance of your due date is advisable (but not before 32 weeks) increasing the amount as you get near or beyond it (from one to no more than three cups). I had a client who swore that she could feel an intensity in her Braxton Hicks contractions whenever she had a cup of raspberry leaf tea. Again, it won't bring on labour if your body is not ready, but it might help to prepare you. It is also nutrient rich and contains good levels of the vitamins A, C, E and B so it is good to drink post-natally as well, to replenish you after the birth. As with anything you want to take in pregnancy, run the idea by your midwife before you start drinking it and don't overdo it.

HAVE SEX

I know having sex is probably the last thing on your mind, or your partner's for that matter. You are as cumbersome and big as you'll ever be and you are being told to somehow also manage sexy! But there are prostaglandins in semen that help soften the cervix in preparation for dilation, and the oxytocin that is produced with nipple stimulation and orgasm can also help to get things started. While not necessarily enticing at this stage, sex is perfectly safe so long as your waters haven't broken. If they have, then it's best not to have sex to avoid any risk of infection. If you really don't feel up to it, then using a breast pump for 20 minutes can stimulate the nipples and in turn release prolactin and oxytocin to help kick-start labour.

EAT A HOT CURRY

There is absolutely no science behind this at all, but some women swear by it. The theory is that because the cervix and the digestive system are connected by the same neural network, stimulating one (a hot curry in the belly) will in turn stimulate the other. If you don't usually eat spicy food, then this is probably not the best time to start foraying into the exotic, but if a good dose of spice is right up your street then there can be no harm in giving it a go. I am sure I could feel the first rumblings of labour with my second child after a particularly fiery tom yum soup!

ACUPRESSURE

There are two pressure points that you can massage after your due date has come and gone, which are said to stimulate the uterus. The first is about three fingers widths above the bony part of the ankle on the inner calf, and the other point is on the 'webbed' bit between your thumb and forefinger. You'll know you've found the points as they are a bit sore when you apply pressure to them. Massage these for several minutes a couple of times a day. Acupuncture is also meant to help stimulate labour, so if it's something you do regularly or you have been having treatments throughout your pregnancy, then you might want to book a trip to your acupuncturist.

ENJOY THE TIME YOU HAVE

As impatient as you might feel, it is equally good to remember that very soon your life is going to change really quite dramatically, and these days in wait will not mean anything once your baby is here. They are, however, a lovely time to do all the things that are about to become much more rare – indulging in long bubble baths, going to the cinema, going out for dinner with your partner. Anything, in fact, that will be harder to do with children in tow. There is a beautiful public garden near where I live that doesn't allow children, so I always say to overdue mothers to go and have a walk in it, or better still pack a picnic and go with your partner for a long lazy lunch. You might feel like you are being incredibly indulgent, but soon you'll have a whole other person to take care of, so enjoy the time to yourself as much as you can.

What is Happening in the Lead-up to Labour?

Waiting for labour to begin can be frustrating, so it might be helpful to know that things will be happening, even if you can't necessarily feel them. During the last few weeks of pregnancy your baby's head will engage in the opening of the pelvis, known as the pelvic inlet. Some women can feel when this happens, and even if you don't feel the process you are likely to feel the impact; you will feel much heavier in the pelvis, might be able to breathe a little more easily and tying your own shoelaces might be within the realms of possibility again, as space is seemingly created in your upper belly. Don't get too excited, though – one downside is that you will probably need to pee more often, as the baby will be exerting more pressure on your bladder and, if you haven't done so already, you will almost certainly start to waddle.

Sometimes a baby will not engage until the very last minute, and this is often the case in second or subsequent pregnancies where there is more room in the uterus for them to play around.

Your midwife will measure how far your baby's head is engaged by dividing the head into fifths and giving you a measurement accordingly. So 5/5 engaged means fully engaged, 3/5 means three-fifths of the head is in the pelvic inlet. Very occasionally a midwife will talk in the reverse so it's worth checking her finding.

Your cervix, which is being held shut by a mucus plug, will also be softening in the week or two leading up to birth. Like a fruit, it is beginning to ripen, all in preparation for dilation. Usually the cervix feels firm and something like the tip of your nose, but as you get closer to labour prostaglandins soften it so that it feels squishy rather than firm. It will also begin to efface, which is just a fancy way of saying thin out. Sometimes your midwife will give you a measurement of this in percentage terms – 0 per cent is not thinned at all and 100 per cent is paper-thin. If your midwife chooses to tell you the measurement, try not to read too much into it. It can change quite quickly.

Finally, you might also feel an increase in Braxton Hicks contractions (sometimes referred to as practice contractions). They are basically mild contractions of the uterus that have been happening throughout pregnancy, but which get stronger in the lead–up to labour. They can sometimes be uncomfortable, but shouldn't be especially painful or intense. You can also get a hefty bout of them after having sex. If you are feeling uncomfortable, then have a warm bath or go for a walk, both of which should help.

SUMMARY

- Remember that a lot is happening in the lead up to labour, even if it is imperceptible.
- Your baby's head will engage and your cervix will soften, all in preparation for your birth.
- You might get an increase in Braxton-Hicks contractions, though it is equally common to feel nothing at all. This doesn't mean, however, that nothing is happening.
- If your due date comes and goes, then try to stay patient. The average first time mother goes into labour five days after her supposed due date, and in France term is 41 weeks.
- There is not a lot you can due to rush the process, though some things might help nudge things along. Try walking, deep squats, having sex, eating hot curries and drinking raspberry leaf tea.
- Whatever you do, try as much as possible to enjoy the time you have, as life is about to change dramatically!

FIRST STAGE OF LABOUR

'Once it starts, there's no turning back: the peaks and troughs of joy, excitement, fear, pain and bliss ahead will be a dramatic prelude to the arrival of your baby and the delicious calm that follows.'

Dr Yehudi Gordon, *Birth and Beyond*

Labour is a continuum, often with no distinct beginning and a blurred end, but it is useful to try to split it into different parts as a way of understanding the intricacies of each stage and to give you some markers – both physical and emotional – on the journey. In fact, an experienced midwife can often tell how far a woman is in her labour by the look on her face and the sounds she is making alone. But, remember, the boundaries between stages are very often blurred. Sometimes a stage can happen so quickly you might think you have missed it altogether and at other times there are pauses within stages, periods often known to midwives as 'rest and relax'. Occasionally a particular stage can go on seemingly forever, while very often a woman might tell you she was unaware of another. Remember, there are as many births as there are babies, so be prepared for the unexpected.

In purely textbook terms, the first stage of labour is considered to be when the cervix dilates from 0 to 10 cm. It can be further split into pre-labour (about 0-3 cm) and then established labour, which is usually the rest. It is vital to make the distinction between labour and pre-labour because if you start clock-watching from the very first rumble, you might get very despondent. Thirty-six-hour labours tend to be mainly made up of pre-labour. And there is a wonderful version of the 'watched kettle never boils' saying which says a 'timed uterus never contracts'. Ignore the clock and arbitrary timelines. Though we talk in stages, only think in them insofar as it reassures you and gives you some guidance.

The very beginning of labour is a synergy between the mother and the baby. No one is absolutely sure of the cue, but it is believed that when the baby's lungs are fully developed it sends a hormonal signal to its mother, which triggers the uterus to begin contracting. This is why trying to force it to happen before you or the baby are ready is very often futile.

It can be very difficult – particularly as a first-time mother, but even second or third time around – to work out if labour has begun or not. By its nature it can be a very stop-start affair, and it is very easy to misread signs. They say that to a man with a hammer everything looks like a nail, and to an overdue mother, every gripe can often feel like a contraction. There are some little signs that might, however, be helpful to look out for.

Often you'll have a burst of energy followed by a period of calm – that proverbial 'calm before the storm' it could be said. A late surge of the nesting instinct is also often a sign that labour is imminent. Nesting happens throughout labour, but if you find yourself 40 weeks and five days pregnant, straddling a tall ladder with a paintbrush in hand, labour is probably not far off!

A little more subtly, women often look as though they are ready for labour, as the hormones give them a certain puffiness to the face – I always say everyone becomes a bit Angelina Jolie, all big lips and swollen cheeks, as though they have just had a quick Botox session. This is usually easier for other people to notice than you – you'll tend to feel swollen anywhere and everywhere and probably won't notice much difference. But in my classes, I can almost always tell who won't be there the next week based on their pout alone!

A bout of diarrhoea, prolonged backache – not unlike period pains – or a great burst of Braxton Hicks contractions can also be a cue that things are hotting up. So can a 'show'. The neck of the cervix is sealed off with a plug of mucus, and a show is when you find – upon an otherwise normal trip to the loo – this plug of mucus, that is generally greeny-grey and can sometimes be tinged with pink, in your knickers. If there is any evidence of bright red blood then you should let your midwife know, but otherwise just carry on as normal, and assume that labour is not far (though still possibly days) away.

Your waters breaking (sometimes known as a breaking of the membranes) is another sign. This can either come as a big gush of water, or can feel simply like an endless pee. But, remember, even if your waters have not broken, you might still be in labour. Your waters breaking is the most flagged, and potentially most dramatic, of all starts to labour depending on where you find yourself, but it is not at all unusual – particularly with a first birth – for the waters to remain intact until well into established labour. It is even possible, and more common than you might think, for the baby to be born in an intact sac. This is known as being born in the caul, and in medieval times was actually considered to be a sign of good luck. Apparently a child born in an intact sac was said to have special gifts, such as clairvoyance, and so auspicious was this way of being born that the sac was often impressed on to paper and then stored away as an heirloom for the child! It is, however, quite rare, so don't get out the flower press. Most women find their waters break just before the second stage of labour. With the waters out of the way, labour has a tendency to really hot up as the pressure between the baby's head and the cervix is increased dramatically, so be prepared for this if it happens to you.

If your waters break before anything else happens, call your midwife and let her know. Also check the colour – if there is a black-ish, green-ish stain to your waters, it could indicate there is meconium in them which can be, but isn't always, a sign of foetal distress.

What Happens during the First Stage?

In very simple terms, the cervix is thinning (effacing) and dilating. So it is going from 'closed' (0 cm dilated and sealed with the mucus plug) to 'open' (10 cm dilated). If you imagine an upside-down pear, then the bulbous bit at the top would be the uterus and the neck of the pear would be the cervix. Pre-pregnancy the uterus is about the size of a pear, but with a full-term baby inside it is about the size of a watermelon. Before dilation begins the cervix needs to thin, which is like the neck of the pear drawing back up on itself. Some or most of the thinning of the cervix is done during pre-labour or even before, with many women going into labour at 2 cm dilated, having never even known that anything was happening, though very strong Braxton Hicks contractions can account for thinning and early dilation.

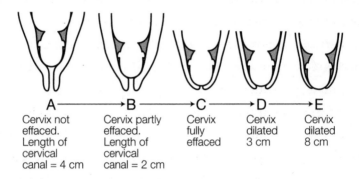

A — Cervix not effaced. Length of cervical canal = 4 cm

B — Cervix partly effaced. Length of cervical canal = 2 cm

C — Cervix fully effaced

D — Cervix dilated 3 cm

E — Cervix dilated 8 cm

Dilation then continues with more obvious contracting of the uterus muscles, as the muscle wall of the uterus tightens. The contractions begin at the top and spread down towards the cervix. The sensation that you feel during labour starts as the tightening begins, peaks when the uterus is fully contracted and then falls away as the uterus releases. With each contraction of the uterus, the cervix is pulled back or opened, which is why dilation is measured. Your midwife will periodically check how far dilated you are (unless you specifically request that she doesn't) with a vaginal examination using her fingers. (See page 29 for more on vaginal examinations.)

It is important that you try to distinguish between pre-labour and labour itself, and I always advise both my yoga class students and my doula clients to ignore labour for as long as possible. And while you can ignore it, it's usually a sign you are in pre-labour rather than established labour. Whatever you do, don't get down on all fours and start breathing heavily the minute you feel your first contraction – otherwise you might find yourself down there for a long time. And maybe don't call all your relatives and friends just yet, as they will then phone constantly checking for updates and driving you mad in the process. Try to just get on with things as normally as possible – albeit with a bit of added excitement and anticipation no doubt; the longer you can just carry on regardless, the better.

If your labour starts during the day, then take yourself off on a walk, watch a funny film or cook yourself a good meal. Make sure you keep hydrated at this stage and eat small but regular meals to keep your energy levels up. On a practical note, it might be an idea to go through your hospital bag one last time, and have it by the door, and check that you have a full tank of petrol in the car. This is often the stage to get your partner home if he isn't there already and arrange for older children to be looked after if that is necessary. If you are planning to have your baby at home, you can also attend to final preparations for your birth space or begin to fill the water pool if you have one. Basically, do anything you like within reason but think of this time as preparation, and the very beginnings of getting into the right head space for birth. Try not to think of yourself as being in full-blown labour until you can't deny it any longer.

If your pre-labour happens at night, then try to get as much rest as possible. Believe it or not it is actually possible to sleep through contractions in early labour. Even if you can't sleep, resist the urge to do too much as you want to get as much rest as possible at this stage. When you're not resting, keep gently mobile to help the baby to get into the best possible position for labour.

Unless your waters have broken or you have reason to believe your labour will be very quick, then you probably don't need to call the hospital just yet – unless of course you are planning a home birth and a midwife will need to come to you. It might be some time yet, but it's a good idea to give her some warning. The same goes for if you have a doula. She won't necessarily need to come to you at this stage, but it will help her plan her day or night ahead if she knows that things might have begun.

There are a number of characteristics of established labour that you can look out for to mark the transition from one to another. The first one is the frequency and length of your contractions. When your contractions start to develop a gentle rhythm, lasting for up to 60 seconds each time and with more even spacing between them – something like five minutes – then you are very likely to be in established labour. At the beginning of labour you will be able to ignore your contractions, but as labour builds they will get much stronger and much more intense, and thereby start to command all of your attention. Another good sign that labour is well established is the behaviour of your stomach when you have a contraction. In very early labour, the shape will not change very much, whereas during established labour your tummy will draw up at the sides and flatten at the top, becoming an almost box-like shape.

Your state of mind is probably the best indicator of your progress. If you are still inclined to go to the phone and have a good old natter to your best friend, you're probably not quite there yet. On the other hand if conversation is becoming more of an inconvenience, this is a wonderful sign that your front brain is beginning to switch off and your primal brain is taking over. Try not to disturb this natural process, but go with it. Turn the lights down low, find a space that you feel instinctively drawn to, surround yourself if necessary with the person or people you would like to have at your birth and remember to breathe fully and deeply. Begin to find mobile and upright positions that feel good, and feel free to experiment with whatever comes naturally.

If you are going to hospital, there is always a question of when you should make the trip. Too early and you risk that your labour has insufficient momentum to withstand the change of scenery. It is not at all uncommon for labour to slow significantly – sometimes

GOOD POSITIONS FOR THE FIRST STAGE

- Walking up and down the stairs.
- Kneeling up and over a beanbag, pile of cushions or birth ball.
- On all fours (with something on the floor to protect your knees).
- Standing in a warm shower with water directed at your pelvis and sacrum.
- Sitting on a birth ball with your legs wide apart, rocking your pelvis back and forward.
- If you need to lie down, lying on your left-hand side with your upper body supported.
- If labour is fast and furious, the knee–chest position (see page 115).

to even stop for a time – when you make the move to hospital. Labouring at home in the early stages, where your surroundings are familiar and you can feel safe and protected, is a good idea as long as you have no complications. On the other hand, you don't want to leave it so late that you are at the peak of your labour on the back seat of the car or worse still, giving birth to a little girl on the M11 hard shoulder! Contractions every three or four minutes, lasting about 90 seconds, is a useful rule of thumb, but seek the advice of your midwife and let your instincts guide you too. You will probably know when it is the right time to go and when you feel like you need the added support of a midwife by your side. If you are giving birth at home, then you have the luxury of being able to stay put, and allow the midwife to come to you.

How to Cope with Established Labour

Occasionally a woman has what she describes as a pain-free birth, and many a midwife will testify to being duped by women who have done hypnobirthing and who do not look as though they are in labour. But I would risk having things thrown at me if I tried to proclaim that birth is always, or even commonly, this way. For the majority of women, it will be hard work: primal, sweaty and challenging. Many women will say they found it painful, but in the same breath they very often assure me that they felt they could cope with the pain, or that the quality of it was not as they expected.

'It wasn't a bad sort of pain,' one woman said to me, 'just a challenging sort.'

'It is the pain of exertion, not of illness,' another woman once said, and her words are echoed by mother after mother.

Birth also has a huge emotional component; you are being asked to draw on every resource you have, to dig deep, and to go to places that you might never have accessed before. It is not at all unusual to completely lose track of time, or to feel like you are on another planet or out of this world. The best thing is to try, as much as possible, to allow yourself to just let go and to let things unfold.

You are also likely to feel every range of emotions imaginable: determination, liberation, strength, despair, weepiness and gratitude. You can oscillate between feeling hot and cold, energetic and exhausted. You might also have bouts of nausea or even throw up (this is sometimes better as it will relieve you of the nausea!)

Remember, giving birth might well be the toughest thing you ever do, but it can be the most fulfilling, most momentous, most confidence-boosting and awe-inspiring thing you ever do,

HOMEOPATHIC HELP DURING LABOUR

- To minimise swelling and bruising – ARNICA 200c under the tongue every 30 minutes.
- To establish strong contractions – CAULOPHYLLUM 200c at the beginning and then every eight hours if necessary.
- To cope with a fast labour – 1 dose of ACONITE 200c.
- To counter back pain – 1 dose of Nat Mur 200c.
- If you are exhausted – 1 dose of KALI PHOS 200c.
- If you are weepy or struggling – 1 dose of PULSATILLA 200c.

too. The odd woman proclaims that she never wants to do it again, yet many more feel robbed if they cannot have the experience another time.

There is a whole spectrum of ways to cope with labour, ranging from a full epidural at one end – now very common in the West – to a simple call-and-response song that is used in Central African Republic where the mother sings 'EI-OH mama ti mbi, ti mbi aso mbi' ('Ei-Oh mother of mine, my belly hurts me') to which the response is 'Kanda be ti MO!' ('Tie up your heart') – in other words, 'Tough it out'!

And along this epidural–tough-it-out spectrum are all manner of ways, many of which have been or will be explored in other chapters; being active (chapter two), having one-to-one support (chapter three) and using water (chapter five).

Now I will take you through a few other ideas that have proved useful to women. Remember, none of this is prescriptive; I know many a mother who has made up her coping mechanism while in labour. The best guide, as always in matters of pregnancy, birth and mothering, is your instincts, but you might want to consider some of the following in advance.

AROMATHERAPY

A lovely, gentle way to help cope with labour, aromatherapy is something you can use at home and hospital alike. This might be a nice time to consider using essential oils. Some people like to burn oils, but in my experience you can like a particular smell one moment but then it makes you feel nauseous the next. It is also usually not possible to bring candles into the hospital.

Placing a few drops on a tissue is a better way to use oils – that way you can have a small sniff as and when you want to, but easily get rid of the smell if it is not having the desired effect. Clary-sage is an especially good oil to use to really get things going, but go very easy – it is very strong and can have quite a powerful impact on your contractions. Put a drop or two on a tissue, breathe the smell in gently and then take it away and see how you feel. Jasmine is also a good birth oil to use, as it is soothing, uplifting as well as renowned for reducing inhibitions – all of which are of great benefit during birth. Jasmine can also boost contractions so, as with all oils, use it sparingly. In fact, both jasmine and clary-sage should not be used before the eighth month of pregnancy and all oils should only be used with the supervision of a midwife. Lavender, rose and neroli are also oils that you might want to consider as they are relaxing and mentally uplifting and can be used safely throughout pregnancy and birth. Make sure you always get the guidance of a trained aromatherapist or that you use the stronger oils under the supervision of your midwife.

Another way of using oils is to make up a massage oil that your birth partner can massage into your sacrum or on to your feet, concentrating particularly on the soft part of your big toes (the site of the pituitary reflex), which helps to initiate efficient contractions.

As well as their physical benefits oils help to create a calm atmosphere, which can be lovely for when you are in labour. Taking a scent with you is also a clever way to create continuity between birthing places, when you make the transition from

ANTICIPATION

Try to stay within your labour as much as possible and to *antic-ipate* the contractions as they come. Think about the way a body surfer catches a wave. If he waited for the wave to be on top of him before he began to swim, he would be caught up in its full force, dumped by the wave, thrown beneath the surface of the water, churned around like a washing machine, and spat back up – probably just in time to have another wave crash on top of him. Instead, a good body surfer will anticipate, swimming just as he begins to feel the swell of the wave behind him, getting one step ahead so that when the wave breaks, he is already there, swimming ahead of it, swept along by its force but not over-whelmed by it. A woman in labour is like that body surfer. As you feel a contraction begin to build, you need to anticipate and begin to move and sway and rotate your pelvis as your instincts guide you. Hum, make noises, sing if necessary. Breathe fully and deeply. You will feel the contraction build, but you are already one step ahead. Your mind is turned inward, you are in your own mental space, and you are moving to help your body cope. Before you know it, the contraction will peak, and just at the point you might think you can't cope, you have – it's gone. Now you can rest, lying forward over a beanbag or a birth ball, or relaxing in the water pool. Feel all the endorphins flood-ing through your body. Contractions are spoken of constantly in birth preparation but what is little spoken of is the space

The rooms you labour in won't look at all alike, but it can be reassuring if they at least smell the same.

home to hospital.

between them. And yet it is this space that not only makes labour bearable but is also, if you are looking out for it, the good bit. Your uterus has worked hard and there is a reward; a wonderful, often soporific, buzzing sensation throughout your body, a literal flooding of endorphins and hormones. If you have anticipated and stayed ahead of the wave, then you will be in the perfect physical and mental state to enjoy this in-between stage, before preparing and moving once more for the next contraction as and when it begins to build. With every contraction think to yourself 'that is one less'. There are a finite number of contractions during any one labour. We – annoyingly – don't know how many there will be, but we can rest assured that it is finite. Every one you have managed is one less that you have ahead of you. Remind yourself of that when a contraction has passed and you are relaxing in the space between them.

BREATHING

I don't think the importance of breathing during labour – as obvious as it sounds – can be underestimated and yet often it is not overly emphasised in antenatal preparation. Breathing effectively is absolutely key to labour. Birth classes over the years have been littered with breathing techniques, with many a doctor becoming famous on the back of a particular piece of advice taking off. The most talked about is probably Dr Lamaze with his various techniques – baseline, slow, blowing, patterned and cleansing. For some women learning these techniques can be a useful distraction and can actually make her breathe properly, but concerns over whether you are getting the technique right or not can often be more confusing than beneficial. It can also keep that front brain more switched on than it should be. So I encourage women to forget techniques and patterns, and just breathe fully and deeply, using an audible sigh, if necessary, to feel the full physical benefits of the exhalation.

It sounds simplistic to just say 'breathe', but it is an instinctive reaction to hold our breath if we are nervous or feel fearful, tightening our jaw and clenching our bodies. And the chances are, if everywhere else is stiff and tight, then your cervix is going to be, too.

Ina May Gaskin talks about maintaining a soft mouth and uses an amusing but also entirely useful analogy, encouraging women to have horse-lips – in public talks she does a wonderful re-enactment of a horse shaking its head and pouting its lips! Breathing out fully and deeply in response to every contraction – and getting your partner to remind you to do so – is simple but hugely effective.

Even better, if you can add some sound to the out breath – a gentle hum, a short mental mantra even – you will find that the mind clears (that is why monks chant to help them meditate) and the body softens. It doesn't have to be wholehearted chanting, but just a gentle hum or audible moan can sometimes help you find and maintain a breathing rhythm.

Keep remembering that every contraction is one that you will never have again, and takes you one step closer to meeting your baby. One mother usefully found herself imagining her labour as a string of beads, and with every contraction a bead fell from the imaginary string. Other mothers have imagined climbing a mountain, with each contraction getting them closer to the top. The image matters less than the feeling of making progress. You might want to think up something prior to labour that might help you, though more often than not the images or ideas will come to you instinctively.

VISUALISATION

A surprisingly powerful tool, visualisation should be part of your 'bag of tricks' for coping with the first and the second stage of labour. It has to a degree been overexposed by the 'new-age' posse, and our intensively rational education makes the majority of us automatic disbelievers. What could imagining myself on a white sandy beach possibly have to do with giving birth to a baby? While the white sandy beach works for some people, others might visualise something more specific. Actually visualising the baby making its spiralling descent through the birth canal can be a very powerful tool. And, remember, the placebo effect is scientific proof of mind over matter, so this does not need to be the preserve of hippy types.

I remember talking to one of my very close friends who was preparing for a natural birth after a Caesarean first time around, with the obstetrician Yehudi Gordon. To say she is not a hippy type is the understatement of the century – anything but. She was reporting back on all of her antentatal preparation and singing its praises, but confessed to a serious discomfort with the visualisations that Yehudi was very keen on. 'I just don't get it,' she would complain to me. 'Everything else he makes me do makes perfect sense, and yet I just can't for the life of me understand how visualising is going to make the smallest bit of difference.' Yet come to her labour and this self-same, non-hippy mother found herself instinctively using these practised images during the birth of her second son – in her case, picturing the baby moving down and through the pelvic canal with every contraction at a time when her labour had seemingly slowed and her baby was taking his time. Against her better judgement and much to her surprise, she now swears that the visualisations made a difference. She could actually feel him move every time she simply pictured him doing so. Proof perhaps that even the greatest non-believers can, it seems, become ardent converts.

Remember, labour will build in intensity over the first stage, so what works for you at a particular moment might be less effective several centimetres down the line. Labour is a process and your feelings – both mental and physical – are likely to change all the time.

Be aware that it is very normal to, at times, feel nauseous during labour, and even to be sick, to feel hot, or cold, and to both laugh and cry. Your midwife will be used to seeing all of this and will not be perturbed, so whatever you are feeling, let it out and try not to worry. As much as possible, go with your labour rather than fighting it at any point. The less you resist or think too much about anything the more likely it is that your labour will progress in the labyrinth-like way that it should.

SUMMARY

- Ignore your labour until you can't any longer.
- Allow the shut-down process to happen. Don't fight the fact that you will want to withdraw, talk less and seek out privacy and darkness as your labour progresses.
- Stay within your labour as much as possible, anticipating each contraction in the same way a body surfer anticipates waves.
- Remember that contractions are not continuous, and the pauses in between them can be amazing. Relax fully between contractions and enjoy the cocktail of hormones flooding through your body.
- Think of every contraction as one less to do. You will never have that contraction again. Every one is a step closer to your baby.
- Keep hydrated with water drunk through a bendy straw, and keep your energy levels up with snacks.
- Breathe fully and deeply – focus especially on the exhalation. Many midwives say it is all in the breathing and can recognise when a woman has done yoga because of the way she breathes.
- Make sounds if necessary – birth is primal and is rarely silent.
- Let go, let go, let go.

TRANSITION

'There is power that comes to women when they give birth. They don't ask for it, it simply invades them. Accumulates like clouds on the horizon and then passes through, carrying a child with it.'

Penny Armstrong and Sheryl Feldman, *A Wise Birth*

The Story of Adrenaline

So you've breathed, moved, rolled and hummed your way through the first stage of labour. It has probably been some time, you might be getting a little tired, but the truth is *you are doing it*. You have climbed three-quarters of the way up the mountain, the summit is not far off and you can begin to smell the change in the air. You are now 8 cm dilated and your contractions are two minutes apart, lasting at least 90 seconds, perhaps a little longer. You are coping, the baby is doing well and your partner has been with you every step of the way. And then you get to the part that is probably the hardest of all – transition. For it would be misleading to say that transition wasn't usually tricky.

At this stage you are almost fully dilated, but not quite. Instead of being well spaced, contractions are now starting to come almost back to back, encouraging the cervix to its final opening. There is little time to recover or to anticipate any more, so you might begin to feel overwhelmed, not by the physical sensations or the pain, but by the fact that you don't seem to have time to catch your breath. It is not unusual to start feeling extremely cold or uncomfortably hot, and some mothers might start shaking at this stage. Often transition is marked in the labour room by a call and response between mother and midwife, with the mother crying out 'I can't do it' and the midwife responding 'But you are … '. Believe her, because it is true. Try not to worry, or to think that there is anything wrong. It might not look or feel like you are doing well, but you are. And, remember, if you can, that this is entirely normal, natural and even – as I will explain – necessary.

If you are unprepared, transition can be really difficult, both for you and for your partner if he hasn't seen it before, but once you understand what is happening, and, crucially, why it is happening, then you can hopefully welcome this stage instead of worrying about it. For, perhaps bizarrely, feeling swamped and fearful at this stage is exactly what is supposed to happen.

All too often we are led to believe that women are somehow badly designed for birth; that their bodies and minds are out of sync and that unlike other animals we just do birth badly. Transition is utter proof that far from being badly designed, we are very well designed, with mind and body working together in almost miraculous harmony.

As we looked at earlier, during the first stage of labour, adrenaline is dreaded enemy number one, so much so that the entire set-up for birth should be designed in an attempt to avoid anything that will create fear in your mind and adrenaline in your body – hence the absolute importance of privacy and security for the first stage.

The reason for adrenaline being so unhelpful during the first stage can be found way back in our evolutionary past, explained by that good old 'fight or flight' system that we so often hear about. Our ancestors would have been exceptionally vulnerable during birth, exposed to countless predators on the plains or in the forest. Adrenaline would have served as their only protective mechanism. If we were giving birth in the wild and found ourselves disturbed by a hungry lion, we would have had to get up and run. Fleeing while heavily pregnant is hard enough, let alone while being in the full throes of labour, so the impact of adrenaline is to stop labour deliberately, shutting down the whole process to give us a chance to get up and run away.

During the second stage of labour, however, adrenaline has the opposite effect. This is when you are past the point of no return – you cannot go anywhere when you have a baby's head between your legs! So to protect you, adrenaline will speed up labour instead of stopping it, making you deliver the baby quick-smart. In theory, you could then pick up the baby and run, lion in hot pursuit. The result of this little in-built mechanism is that during the second stage, far from being a hindrance a good burst of adrenaline is helpful, even necessary. And it isn't just necessary for you. The adrenaline induces stress in the baby, stimulating his survival instinct and his lungs in preparation for breathing at birth. Contrary to what we might think, the stress of birth actually serves a very positive purpose, for both mother and baby alike.

Obviously it is impossible to deliberately orchestrate this physiological change in the context of a normal birth, where lions are unlikely to feature. But we don't need lions. Instead we have a little in-built dose of mental magic. Or 'transition'. Back-to-back contractions that are difficult and overwhelming naturally make a mother – even one who has been coping remarkably until then – feel fearful. It doesn't need to last long; a fleeting dose of fear is enough for your body to produce adrenaline, which takes you automatically and usually seamlessly into the second stage of labour. In other words, it has the effect that a lion would have had on the prairie in prehistoric times. The body produces back-to-back contractions that affect the mind, making it fearful. The mind in turn produces adrenaline, which at this point makes the body give birth quick-smart. Body affects mind – mind affects body. Just like magic.

So as much as possible, try to simply breathe through this stage, and remind yourself that it is entirely normal and natural and that it won't last long. Even more importantly, remember it is bringing you one giant step closer to meeting your baby. Make sure your partner knows all about transition so that instead of feeling worried, he can simply offer you quiet words of reassurance and do so convincingly.

SUMMARY

- Transition is the hardest part of labour for most women. You are likely to feel overwhelmed, vulnerable and out of control.

- It is normal, even necessary, for you to find transition difficult. It is also an example of how finely tuned the body and mind are for birth.

- It is not uncommon to start shaking, to throw up and to feel extremely hot or cold. You will also probably feel very thirsty.

- Transition will pass. It is too late at this stage to take any pain relief, though it might be just the moment you want it.

- Transition is designed to produce the adrenaline that is necessary to bring your baby into the world.

- Rest assured it will not be long till you meet your baby.

SECOND STAGE OF LABOUR

'Breathe
help me as the next generation carves a pathway from my body.
Breathe
in this space between worlds I link my life and yours.
Breathe
each physical exertion pushes you towards my arms.
Breathe
in vigour and action.'
Maori poem by Roma Potiki

The second stage of labour is markedly different from the first, primarily because adrenaline is present in huge amounts, coursing through your veins, bringing you back from that 'other planet' and transforming you into an energised, enlivened, primal animal. Whereas before you might well have wanted to keep your clothes on during the first stage, now you will be more likely to want to rip them off. Whereas in the first stage you might have moaned quietly to yourself, humming or singing your way through contractions, now the sounds of the labour room will be altogether more animal-like: growls and roars. In fact, I often liken a mother in the second stage to a lioness – big, strong and noisy.

What is Happening?

In purely textbook terms, the second stage of labour is when the cervix has completely dilated and the baby is out of the uterus and descending through the birth canal, passing through the perineum and coming out into the world. The contractions feel markedly different, tending to be described as less painful but more intense, still 60 to 90 seconds long but often spaced much further apart – back to between three and five minutes. It is common to feel what is described as an 'urge to push' at this stage – an irresistible bearing down, which comes from the descent of the baby's head on the muscular pelvic floor. It can, first time around, feel as though the baby might just be coming out of your bottom – rest assured she is not!

If, prior to feeling this 'urge to push', you experience a pause in the proceedings do not be alarmed. This is not uncommon and is often referred to as the 'rest and be thankful' stage, with some midwives arguing that it is a period when the uterus is readjusting itself and the baby is potentially getting into its final position ready for birth. While such pauses are normal in the context of a natural labour (experienced midwives say another one often occurs at 6 cm dilation), less-experienced midwives and doctors who want labour on a plottable course, and who are loath to sit on their hands, can sometimes be unnerved by the need to wait. But as long as you and your baby are okay and your baby is regularly monitored, there should be no cause for concern. Patience, as they say, is a virtue and can be particularly so at this stage of labour.

An Anterior Lip

Most women have fully dilated by the time they get the urge to push, but very occasionally you might have an anterior lip. This is a little section of the cervix in front of the baby's head that for one reason or another has not yet dilated with the rest of the cervix. Sometimes a midwife can literally push it out of the way, though more often it is a matter of waiting for several more contractions and resisting (easier said than done) the urge to bear down. The best way to do this is to adopt the 'knee–chest' position (see page 115), with your chest on the bed or the floor and your bottom in the air. As you feel a contraction, try to pant or gently blow rather than bear down. After a series of contractions, the cervix should have completely dilated.

The 'Urge to Push'

When it comes, everyone experiences the second stage slightly differently. Some women feel no need to push but more a need to simply let go and allow their body to open for the baby. This often happens in the case of a truly natural birth where a woman is experiencing what Michel Odent describes as a 'foetal ejection reflex'.[29] This, he says, is an involuntary and intuitive pelvic thrust that a woman performs spontaneously in response to the huge surge of adrenaline that comes with transition. Instead of squeezing and straining, a mother who is experiencing such a second stage just needs to follow her body's cues and completely let go.

Other women feel the need to be part of the process of birthing the baby and need to harness their energy, aiding the descent by bearing down or actively pushing with each contraction. If you can, it is good to remain upright and supported at this stage to harness the help of gravity and to be in a position that opens the pelvis to its maximum. Many woman instinctively lean forward, which is believed to be the best position for protecting the perineum. Rather than pushing noisily from the throat or mouth, focus as much as possible on bearing down through the pelvis and internalising any sounds you feel compelled to make. Putting your chin to your chest or pushing into your bottom to direct your energy are two much-used techniques. It is also important to wait for a contraction before you push. Try to really work with your body at this stage. And really listen to your midwife as she will help you co-ordinate your efforts with your contractions so that you do not use up unnecessary energy. Try to keep any noises you do make gravelly and low – good primal sounds to open the body. By all means make them – this is not the time to be meek and self-conscious. You are giving birth and it is a big, almighty act. Let it be.

GOOD POSITIONS FOR THE SECOND STAGE

- Standing in an upright and supported squat.
- On all fours.
- Kneeling with one leg raised (and holding either your partner or edge of the bed).
- Sitting on a birth stool.
- Upright and leaning over the back of the bed or a pile of cushions.
- Upright, squatting in a pool.

Having some control over your pelvic floor can be of great benefit during this stage and, quite apart from all the other benefits, is
a good reason to have been practising your pelvic floor exercises
(see below), so you are more likely to be able to actively relax
them for the second stage.

PELVIC FLOOR EXERCISES

The pelvic floor is a band of muscles that runs in a figure of
eight around the vagina and the anus. These muscles work
to keep your uterus and other organs in place, and perform a
vital role in helping the rotation of the baby through the birth
canal. As pregnancy progresses and through the course of the
birth process, they obviously come under some pressure so
it is important to do pelvic floor exercises to keep them functioning optimally. The penalty for not doing it is the rather
charming habit of peeing when you laugh or sneeze, a
slightly duller sex life, the possibility of a longer second stage
and, in the worst-case (but thankfully rare) scenario, uterine
prolapse – none of which you should have to deal with.

These problems can be avoided, for the most part, by
regularly doing pelvic floor exercises before and after the
birth. Sounds simple, but the problem is for most women it
is nigh on impossible to remember to do them. I suggest a
post-it note above the sink or on the mirror in the bathroom,
so you'll remember to do them at least twice a day, when
you brush your teeth.

Start by locating the muscles: the next time you go to the toilet, stop peeing mid-stream. The muscles you contract to do this are your pelvic floor. There are three different types of exercises you can do, and my advice is to do a mixture of all three, and increase the amount you do each time as you develop strength and control in the muscles.

The first is a simple tightening and then releasing, which you can do up to 20 times.

The second type is where you tighten the pelvic floor, hold for up to five seconds and then release, which you can do between five and 10 times every session.

And the third type is known as the 'elevator' where you try to draw up on the pelvic floor in stages, as though you are going up in a lift. As you develop more control, you might find that you can also come back down in stages, too.

If you find pelvic floor exercises difficult at first, don't worry. The muscles develop tone and are much easier to locate very quickly, so persevere and just work towards as many sessions a day as you can manage.

Don't be surprised or alarmed if, as your baby descends, it feels as though it retreats after each contraction. Think of it as taking two steps forward and then one back, but remember that still means you are making progress. The baby's descent is opening your body. If it's your first baby, it is doing it for the first time, and the body will naturally be resistant but, rest assured, it is opening with every contraction. Believe that it can open – because it can and will – and that it is doing so even if your progress seems slow.

The birth of your baby's head through the perineum, known as crowning, is accompanied by a momentary burning or stinging sensation. This is much reduced by the use of water, but be reassured that on dry land it does not last very long. Really listen to your midwife again at this stage, as she might well encourage you to simply pant rather than push as a way of easing your baby as gently as possible through the perinuem. A perineum softened by regular massage leading up to the birth will stretch more readily and easily (see below) and is very worthy preparation.

PERINEUM MASSAGE

Perineum massage is advised from about 34 to 36 weeks of pregnancy to increase the elasticity of the perineum to enable it to stretch better during labour. Scientific research is ambivalent about its benefits but anecdotal stories tend to be very positive. As it won't hurt to do it, it's surely worth a try.

Many books advise you to get your partner to give you the massage. As it's possibly the least sexy thing you could ask for, I suggest you do it yourself. The choice as to who is chief masseur is, however, entirely up to you!

You will need unscented massage oil, available in any health food shop, a mirror (optional) and privacy. Wash your hands and make sure your nails aren't too long. Sit in a warm comfortable area, spreading your legs apart in a semi-sitting birthing position, or lift one leg up – a closed toilet can be a useful prop. To become familiar with the perineal area, you can use a mirror for the first few massages. Put oil on your thumb and forefinger, and then put your thumb into your vagina, making sure you don't go in too far. Begin to massage the area, alternating between rubbing the perineum tissue between your thumb and forefinger, and applying gentle pressure with the thumb, drawing the perineum down until you feel a slight burning sensation. Be gentle.

Do this several times a week from 34 weeks, and daily from about 36 weeks, working for between three and five minutes each time. You will find that very quickly the area begins to feel thinner and more elastic. This will obviously help the area stretch more easily, but should also crucially give you the confidence that you can stretch comfortably during the second stage of labour.

Putting your hand down to feel your baby's head as it crowns can be a lovely way to focus your efforts, and often a midwife will offer to use a mirror to show you your baby emerging.

Once your baby's head is through, you will feel an almost immediate relief. Often there is a pause and a wait for a few minutes before the rest of your baby is born with the next contraction. The feeling you will have then is indescribable; a heady mix of relief, wonder, awe and emotion. You might laugh or cry or do both. Whatever you do, seeing your baby for the first time will be something you are unlikely to ever forget and is pure testament to the adage that the hardest things in life are often the best.

Your Baby

Don't be at all surprised if your baby is born a little blue – he will turn a normal pink colour as soon as breathing is established. Remember that until the cord stops pulsating he is still being fed oxygen through the placenta. He will also be covered in a creamy substance called vernix, which helps to protect against the inevitable change in temperature experienced at birth. The head can also sometimes be a strange shape, particularly after a prolonged second stage, but it is designed to mould and will shift back into place over the coming days and weeks. Whatever the intricacies of how your baby looks, pink, and wrinkled and slippery, you are still likely to think he is the most beautiful thing you have ever seen.

SUMMARY

- Understand, at least intellectually, what to expect by reading, going to classes and talking to your midwife.
- Be upright, enabling gravity to assist you.
- Be willing to let go. The second stage of labour is in every sense an act of letting go, both mentally and physically. Prudery has no place in the labour room at this stage, so be willing to really lose yourself to the process. It is natural and normal and an extraordinary thing. You are giving birth.
- Listen to your midwife. Whereas during the first stage a good midwife is one who allows labour to unfold, during the second stage her advice and support can be invaluable. She can ensure that your baby's entry into the world is as gentle as possible on you both. Unless, of course, it is a true foetal ejection reflex, where a quiet midwife is all that is necessary.
- Allow yourself to make sounds, but try to contain as much as you can and keep any sound you do make low and primal sounding.
- Breathe down into your bottom and take your chin to your chest.
- Visualise the baby descending through the pelvic canal. Remember you are moments away from meeting.

THIRD STAGE AND THE HOUR AFTER BIRTH

'For the new mother, the third stage is a time of reaping the rewards of her labour.'
Sarah Buckley, *Gentle Birth, Gentle Mothering*

When mothers come back to tell their birth stories, more often than not they finish with the actual birthing of their babies. While this understandably feels like the pinnacle, labour is not yet over. The placenta needs to come away from the uterus wall and be born as well.

The Placenta

The placenta is an extraordinary thing. It is a temporary organ, and serves as no less than the baby's lifeline for nine months in the womb, performing many of the functions that the baby will undertake for himself in those early minutes of life outside the womb – breathing, excreting and digesting. When you first find out you are pregnant, your uterus contains little more than a cluster of cells. Half of those go on to become your baby, and the other half, the placenta. So when other cultures refer to the placenta as the baby's twin, they are being more scientific than they probably realise!

The placenta is attached on one side to the uterus with finger-like tissues called villi, and on the other side to the baby by the umbilical cord, which, by the time your baby is born, has grown to up to a metre in length. Its role is essential, providing both oxygen and nutrients from your bloodstream to your baby's (and more or less anything else you consume, hence why toxins should be kept to a minimum during pregnancy). This vital role is recognised in other cultures and the placenta is often subject to great ritual and symbolism.

The most beautiful I have heard of is in New Zealand, where a place is chosen after the birth of the baby for the placenta to be buried – that is then considered to be the baby's sacred or special place, somewhere that he might return to again and again, a sort of second home. In other places the placenta is planted beneath a tree, used to provide inspiration for prints and drawings, and is even sometimes consumed by the mother and her family in a quest to access its supposed nutritious and anti-depressant qualities.

More often than not in the West, rituals are bypassed and the placenta is considered little more than clinical waste, thrown out with all the other hospital rubbish. In all likelihood, the hospital you give birth in will assume that you will have no attachment to your placenta, so by all means if you would like to do something more interesting with it, then speak up. Some people find it fascinating to see how this quite extraordinary organ functions and most midwives will be more than happy to show you.

After your baby is born there will be a pause, somewhere between five and 30 minutes. At some point during this time, the placenta will detach from the uterus wall, which you might notice with a cramping feeling or mild contractions. The midwife might note a renewed flush of blood, which will indicate to her that the separation has occurred. You might also feel a heaviness at the base of the uterus, which is the placenta sitting there. In those cases, it will take little more than standing up or getting on your knees for the placenta to come out. Sometimes, you will feel several more contractions, usually not nearly of the magnitude of your earlier ones, and will need to bear down gently, either breathing into your bottom again as you did in the second stage or gently as though breathing into a bottle. Even if you need to help the process along, it shouldn't be too difficult – the placenta is slippery and malleable, so should be birthed with very little effort on your part.

It is essential to recognise that until the placenta is out and has been checked over by a midwife, the birth is not over, and that all the conditions that are conducive to a positive experience during the first and second stage of labour are still relevant to the third. So keep the room dimly lit, quiet and make sure you have no one there who is not completely necessary – which means that relatives and celebrations are best delayed just a little while longer! It is also really important to keep both yourself and the baby warm. If the baby is interested in suckling, then encourage him gently to do so as this will help with the delivery of the placenta. In fact, rather beautifully, your baby's needs and your own are completely aligned at this stage. Your baby needs nothing more than warmth, skin-to-skin contact and gentle nurture. In time he will also need to suckle, and will indicate this with an entirely instinctive rooting around and nuzzling towards the breast. At this stage, your needs are to deliver the placenta safely and have your uterus clamp down to stem the blood flow from the placental site. Both of these are encouraged by your baby's suckling, which produces waves of oxytocin and more contractions. Whoever said Mother Nature wasn't clever?

Managed versus Natural Third Stage

There is some debate as to whether this third stage needs to be managed or not. In most cases, the baby's suckling and your patience will be enough and the placenta will be born in its own time, with just a little help on your part with pushing it out if necessary. The benefits of simply waiting and having a natural third stage is that it gives you the time to leave the umbilical cord intact until it stops pulsating, which ensures the baby gets the last of all the very nutritious blood from the placenta and cord.

Studies have shown that newborns whose umbilical cords are clamped between one and three minutes after pulsation stops have much higher iron levels and therefore less incidence of anaemia than infants whose cords are clamped immediately after delivery.[30]

If you delay clamping, you also leave the placenta as a potential back-up system or breathing safety net, as it continues to provide oxygen through the umbilical cord while your baby establishes his own breathing. Most babies breathe unaided as soon as they are born, and if they don't then there is always help at hand, but by keeping the umbilical cord intact and the placenta attached, it can serve as a back-up in those rare cases that breathing is not immediate.

Despite these benefits, management of the third stage is increasingly common. In a managed third stage, the cord is clamped and cut almost immediately, and then you will be given an injection of syntometrine, which induces immediate and strong contractions in the uterus. This helps with the expulsion of the placenta and the closing down of the placental site. There is no doubt that management has its benefits: the third stage is quicker and there is a reduced risk of blood loss, as the uterus clamps down tightly. It is also advisable to consider a managed third stage if your labour has been exceptionally long. As with all interventions, however, there are not benefits without the inevitable pitfalls. Not only does it mean that the cord tends to be cut early, but the injection can make you feel sick or dizzy and it also increases the risk of a retained placenta, which although uncommon requires manual extraction in the operating theatre under anaesthetic (usually a spinal block).

There does seem, increasingly, to be a middle way on offer, where mothers are asking for a wait-and-see approach – as long as labour has gone well and the baby has been born without too much intervention, the cord is allowed to stop pulsating naturally and there is an allotted amount of time for the placenta to come of its own accord. If it comes and there is no excessive bleeding then the injection is not needed, though if there is evidence of bleeding or a significant delay in the placenta coming out, the injection can be used. If you have any strong feelings either way, it is really important to discuss your options with your midwife and include your preferences in your birth plan (see page 54).

Birth and Bonding

Whatever choices you make regarding the third stage, remember that this is a really special time. You have just met your baby for the first time, and you and your newborn are filled to the brim with oxytocin, making you both absolutely primed for bonding. And because of the adrenaline shot in the second stage, both your pupils and those of your baby will be dilated, compelling you both to stare at one another. Coupled with another stroke of genius on the part of Mother Nature, the fact that your baby can see from the crook of your arm to your eyes, and no further, means that you are both perfectly equipped to simply sit and stare at one another, beginning what will ideally become a process of strong attachment.

Human bonding is complex. Mammals bond almost entirely instinctively – if a sheep has an epidural, it will refuse to suckle its young. Thankfully, we bond through a mixture of hormones and experience. Adoptive mothers fall in love with their babies, and mothers who have had a Caesarean, and therefore have not been exposed to any of the love hormones of birth, are still more than capable of bonding with their children. But there is no doubt that the hours after birth are a sensitive period and have the potential to lay foundations for a relationship that will only continue to grow over the coming days, weeks and months. It makes complete sense to protect this period and allow the mother, father and baby as much time and privacy as possible. Daddy is not left out of this oxytocin love-in – studies have shown that when a father attends the birth of his child, his oxytocin levels rise as well!

Keep the door shut for as long as you can without offending the relatives. Turn the lights down low and enjoy this period of calm. There is no doubt you've earned it, and that you will look back on those first few hours as being really quite magical.

Sometimes, there is a concern over the baby or mother that means the first few hours are interrupted in some way. Do not despair. If you need medical attention, then it might be a lovely time for daddy or another relative to have some precious moments with the baby – if your partner is willing to be skin-to-skin with the baby, then so much the better. If the baby needs attention of some sort, then simply use all the same ideas – skin-to-skin, the nurture of touch and breastfeeding (which also gives you both a lovely oxytocin boost) to more than make up for any lost time.

It cannot be underestimated how important time is when it comes to bonding. For some mothers it is love at first sight, while for others the process is a little slower. Bonding in some women starts before the birth – I know one woman who found herself overwhelmed by the feelings she had for her baby as soon as he had taken his first breath. She couldn't believe that here was a veritable stranger whom she already knew; without any shadow of doubt, she would have stepped in front of a car to save him. Other perfectly sane, heartfelt and emotional women confess to having felt very little other than protective until their toddler was able to speak to them, and engage them in conversations that then had them smitten. There is, of course, no right or wrong on this path of love. Neither ultimately becomes the better mother, but for everyone time is crucial. As one lovely woman in my class wrote to me:

'I remember what you told us about bonding, how it needn't happen right away. I now feel that the process must have begun long before the birth – every time I was chased up the road by a pushy Audi driver, and I wanted to get out and shout at him for putting my baby at risk, or every time I felt a bit ropey and had to take a minute to ask the bump if everything was alright (the bump was always alright, and as a result, so was I). So when the moment came, there was no ooh, aah fireworks. The bond was already there, slowly burning away under all the fuss and the practicality. I already knew how I felt.'

SUMMARY

- The birth is not over until the placenta has been safely born, so it is important to maintain all the same conditions as during the rest of labour – quiet, dim lighting, few people and minimal distraction.
- Decide whether you would like to have a managed or natural third stage, remembering that it is preferable to delay the cutting of the umbilical cord where possible.
- Encouraging the baby to suckle will help with the delivery of the placenta.
- These first few hours after birth are a really special time for you all, so be sure to keep it as undisturbed as possible.
- Remember, bonding is a process and may not happen instantly. Give yourself the time and the space to get to know each other.

CHAPTER 8

Caesareans
When Nature Falters

'You can't just let nature run wild.'
Walt Disney

In my classes, I have often drawn an analogy between a labouring woman and an experienced sailor. A sailor, well versed in the ways of the sea, will learn all he can about navigation, will practise the art of the knot, and understand sails and how to manipulate them. He will have learned to harness the elements, using wind and water to his own end. But a good sailor will always maintain a healthy respect for nature and her vagaries. He will accept that she can be unruly and that she ultimately can preside. The same might be said of a mountaineer. He may well play cat and mouse with the elements, but the mountaineers who succeed in achieving super-human feats are the ones that never let their egos misguide them into thinking nature can be controlled. This delicate balancing act between control borne out of knowledge and surrender to nature is one that should be played out by the pregnant mother.

One of the most common things women who have good experiences come back to me and say is, 'I am so glad I remained

....

open-minded.' It is rare that birth follows our plans to the letter. Sometimes it is as simple as a pool not being ready in time when a water birth was planned, or that a woman opts for an epidural when she thought she wouldn't. (Though perhaps, surprisingly, it is often the other way round – that a woman stipulated she might want an epidural, but then copes better than she imagined.) But, occasionally, the birth goes more dramatically off course, and a baby is born by Caesarean section to a mother who dutifully planned for a natural birth.

For the truth is, with all the good will, planning, hip gyrating and deep breathing in the world, and even armed with a doula, a fabulous midwife and the most perfect environment possible, nature can still throw you a curve ball.

Something might come upon us in the last weeks of pregnancy – persistent placenta praevia (which is when your placenta persistently lies too near or even over the cervix), gestational diabetes or pre-eclampsia, for example – or you might have done some of the hard work but for one reason or another things haven't progressed as they should, leading to an emergency Caesarean.

Either way, remember it is unlikely that you'll need a Caesarean – 90 per cent of women shouldn't need any intervention at all. If you do, however, it is worth knowing it is an incredibly safe alternative to a natural birth.

Whatever you are planning, an open mind in the face of labour can only be a good thing. No matter how much you might want a particular type of birth, doggedly holding on to your birth plan and chastising yourself if you don't follow it to the letter is fruitless. All too often women will report their birth experience back to me, unable to accept the way things went. I know someone who had a Caesarean for placenta praevia and five years on still feels short-changed, even though in that situation there was no other way out for her baby. Your experience of birth is paramount, but so too is the health of both yourself and your baby.

Getting Your Head Around a Caesarean

While there is obviously less you can do to prepare yourself for a Caesarean section, having a sense of what might happen and how you can help yourself through both the experience and the recovery can mean the difference between a good and a bad experience. Faced with anomalies and complications, some women might well be happy to just hand themselves over, but others still feel like they want to a play a part and have a say, in which case there are details that you can request to make the experience a more personal one.

A Short History

There is a myth – the world of birth is littered with them it seems – that Julius Caesar was the first person to be born by Caesarean, hence the name for the operation. The truth is far more complex (and tedious, so I won't bore you with the details), but had much more to do with Roman law than it did with the naturally born Julius and his surviving mother. Early Caesareans were decidedly hit-and-miss affairs, although there are amazing stories of farmers who saved the life of both their wife and child with rudimentary kitchen table surgery! In fact, the first documented Caesarean can be traced as far back as 1588 and was performed by a Swiss pig farmer on his wife after a very protracted and prolonged labour. Not only did Mrs Elizabeth Alespachin and her baby survive, but the job was done so well that she went on to have six more children, including one set of twins. And if that were not surprising enough, her Caesarean-born child went on to defy the life expectancy of that era and lived to the ripe old age of 77!

Medical advances – in the world of anaesthesia, antibiotics and surgery – over the last century have ensured that the Caesarean is now not only a very safe operation but also by far the most common performed on women across the globe. In fact, there are now more women who have Caesareans than people who have their tonsils removed.

One of the most important developments in the history of the Caesarean has been in the change in the incision or, in layman's terms, the 'cut'. Initially the cut was done vertically, leaving a weaker and much more unsightly scar that ran from the belly button to the pubic bone. But then in the early 1900s an alternative cut was developed and gradually perfected. Now known as the bikini cut, because a bikini can – in theory be worn without the scar showing, the incision is much smaller and is a transverse cut just above the pubic bone, usually just below the pubic hairline. Not only is it much more aesthetically pleasing, but it also heals as a much stronger scar, making rupture during subsequent births much less likely.

No doubt, the operation is still major abdominal surgery and your recovery plans should respect this, but medical developments have meant that in most of the Western world women who are faced with the operation should feel in safe hands.

Preparing Yourself

There is obviously a limit to what you can actively do when it comes to having your baby by Caesarean, but it is important to request anything that might mean a lot to you. You might still want your partner to cut the cord, or to announce the sex of the baby. Asking not to be separated from your baby except in an emergency is also a perfectly legitimate request, as is the desire to be skin-to-skin with your baby as soon as she is born. You might also want to ask for there to be silence at the moment of birth so that the first voice the baby hears is yours or your partner's.

Although most Caesareans are undertaken in brightly lit rooms, with quite a number of people in attendance, there are moves among some surgeons to try to make the birth as intimate as possible – in fact, a pioneering Professor Fisk has started a practice that he calls 'the skin-to-skin Caesarean' or 'walking the baby out'. Instead of priding himself on the speed between incision and birth, he wanted to make the experience as close to a natural birth as possible. Parents are encouraged to watch the birth of their baby, and immediate skin-to-skin contact is also encouraged.

In most hospitals, the experience is more standardised, but rest assured that the medical staff looking after you will in all likelihood be incredibly gentle and kind, and will absolutely have the best interest of you, your partner and your baby at heart.

The Standard Procedure

While the details may differ from place to place, it is probably useful to go through a standard Caesarean to give you an idea of what is likely to happen. Of course there are no hard-and-fast rules, but most experiences will go along the following lines. There will come a time when a Caesarean is deemed necessary, which might well be in advance of labour and scheduled (because of a flagged complication) – this is known as an elective Caesarean, even when you haven't exactly chosen it. Alternatively, it can happen within the context of a labour that has faltered and this is known as an emergency Caesarean, which can make it sound more dramatic than it actually is. If you have been in labour, be prepared for the atmosphere to change quite dramatically – the operating theatre is a very different place to all but the most insensitive of delivery rooms. The room will be very brightly lit and necessarily sterile, and instead of just being attended to by a single or maybe two midwives, there will be a whole team of people. As a friend once said, 'I had no idea quite how many people would be in the room. It was practically enough for a football team.'

As well as your partner and yourself, there will be about eight other people in the room if there are no complications. The team will include a midwife, a surgeon, the doctor's assistant, an anaesthetist, the anaesthetist's nurse, a scrub nurse (who helps the doctor with all the instruments) and one or two theatre nurses.

Sometimes there is also a paediatrician on hand and a medical student or two.

You will be asked to sign a consent form, which lists all the complications that could arise from the anaesthesia and the operation, and it's a bit like the leaflet inside a packet of painkillers in that it lists every possible eventuality no matter how unlikely. You will then be given a theatre gown to wear, which is usually one of those beautiful shades of insipid green and open at the back. You will need to take everything off (including jewellery – but not your wedding ring, which will probably be taped – glasses or lenses and hair clips, etc) and just wear the gown. You might well also be given long, tight white socks like the type people sometimes wear on long-haul flights, to reduce your risk of deep-vein thrombosis or blood clots. Either way, you won't look a picture for your photos, but I promise it won't matter!

You will then be taken into theatre, and your partner will be asked to remain outside while you are anaesthetised. Except for serious emergencies, most Caesareans are now performed with either an epidural or a spinal anaesthesia. Both work in the same way in their numbing of the lower half of the body, but differ in terms of where in the spine they are injected.

You will generally be asked to lie on your side or sit on the edge of the operating table leaning over to curl your spine. The anaesthetist will first insert a local anaesthetic (this will feel like a pin prick) and then will give you the epidural or spinal – because of the local anaesthetic you feel nothing at all at this stage. You are then helped on to your back again, and you should feel your abdomen and legs begin to go numb almost immediately. It can be – but isn't always – very strange!

A drape is then hung over your upper belly to create a screen between you and your belly. You will have your pubic hair shaved and a catheter inserted. The shaving is to clear a space for the incision, though a beautician advised that if you know you are having a Caesarean in advance it is best to get waxed as the re-growth is better! The catheter is inserted to keep your bladder (which lies very close to the uterus) empty throughout the oper-ation, and to drain off urine because you will no longer feel the sensation of needing to pee.

Once you are prepped and ready, your partner will be allowed in to be at the head of the table with you. Having someone there to hold your hand and reassure you can be extraordinarily helpful as this is often the most nerve-racking part of the operation. I know women who have had doulas expressly for a Caesarean, and in particular for support at this point, when the anticipation is at its most heightened. Rest assured, from this point it is no more than half an hour before you meet your baby.

When your partner is in, and settled, the anaesthetist will test whether you can feel anything by prodding or gently pricking your belly or leg. Once it is established that you can't feel anything, the surgeon will begin. Your tummy will be painted with antiseptic solution and then the surgeon will do the first incision through the abdomen wall, and the next through the uterus. In a matter of moments, the baby will then be helped out. Although you will feel no pain, you will feel some pressure or a tugging sensation – it feels a little bit like someone is doing the washing-up in your belly, or rummaging around in search of a sock! Whatever the analogy, it should be pressure rather than pain that you are feeling. Again it can be a little strange, but shouldn't be too alarming.

You can, if you wish, ask for the drape to be lowered at this point so that you can see the point of birth through the abdomen, which many couples say is quite a magical moment. Even if it is not as nature intended, it is still the birth of your child and is still both extraordinary and emotional. You could also at this point ask for your partner to announce the sex, or for voices to be hushed so that yours is the first voice your baby hears.

The cord will then be clamped and cut, and then the baby will either be handed directly to you, or will be quickly checked over and have her airways suctioned a little on a table nearby, before being wrapped up and placed in your arms. You should be very much awake, but if by chance you are feeling a little woozy or nauseous (which can sometimes be a side-effect of the anaesthesia), then your partner can take the baby for you. As with a natural birth, having skin-to-skin contact at this stage is a lovely practice and of great benefit to the baby.

Back on the delivery table, you will have your placenta and membranes removed and the surgeon will then begin the process of stitching you up. This tends to take longer than the delivery of the baby, but usually you will barely notice it as you have something rather wonderful to grab your attention! The whole operation tends to take about 45 minutes from start to finish.

When the surgery is complete, you will be taken to a recovery room so that you can be observed for a period before you are taken to the postnatal ward. So long as everything is okay, your baby and your partner will be with you at all times. You will find that a spinal anaesthesia takes about two to three hours to wear off, and an epidural about six to eight.

Recovering from a Caesarean

It can take a little longer to recover from a Caesarean than from a natural birth, but as with all things the experience differs in every circumstance and with every mother. Some women are up and about and entertaining their family at home within a week, while others feel tired and a little sore for much longer. Whichever camp you fall into, remember you have had major abdominal surgery and you need to give your body time to heal. Even if it goes against your nature to do so, try to take things slowly at first. It is better to rest when friends and family are on hand and offering help, rather than to get back to normal too soon only to find that you are worn out six weeks down the line when everyone else is leaving you alone. Whatever you do, don't feel in the least bit guilty about asking for help. Most people, when they undergo major operations, don't have a newborn baby to look after.

You will be encouraged by the midwives on the postnatal ward to get up and move around gently within 24 hours of your operation and it is at around the same time that your catheter will be removed. This will keep your circulation moving and will help with your recovery. Make sure you tell the midwives if you feel dizzy or uncomfortable. Thanks to modern pain relief, there is no reason to be in undue discomfort but your scar will be sore and it is not uncommon to feel referred pain in the back or shoulders. As the effects of the anaesthetic wear off, you will be offered other pain relief in the form of capsules or suppositories. If you don't feel as though you are getting enough, then speak up. The midwives are there to help you, but they can't second-guess how you are feeling.

Even with pain relief, you might find it uncomfortable for the first few days and possibly weeks if you laugh, cough or sneeze – so maybe don't invite any funny friends over for a while! If they do pitch up, gently hold your scar or hold a pillow across it if you need to laugh, and the same goes for coughing and sneezing. It is also more comfortable if you wear bigger clothes than usual – tracksuit bottoms with a gentle elasticated waist or pyjama bottoms, and bigger than usual knickers. It will need to be function before fashion for a little longer, I'm afraid.

Your scar will be surprisingly small, though it can be a bit angry and red at the beginning. Keep an eye on it for signs of infection – extra soreness or redness and any pussy discharge – over the coming days and weeks, and if you see anything you are not sure about, then just let your midwife know. She will be checking you regularly for the duration of your stay in hospital, which will be up to three or four days depending on how mobile you feel. Usually the stitches are dissolvable; otherwise they will be removed by a nurse after a week or so. It is not at all unusual for your scar to feel itchy as it heals (remember scabs on your knees as a child?), and it can also feel numb for up to 12 weeks or so. Rest assured that within several months to a year, all that will be left is a faint line and all sensation will have returned.

In just the same way as after a natural birth, it is normal for you to bleed after the birth (known as lochia) and so sanitary pads in your big knickers are a good idea. All very unglamorous, I know!

As well as medicated pain relief, it is useful to have a little suitcase of alternative remedies at your disposal to help with your recovery. Homeopathy can be a real help – Arnica is a godsend for bruising, as is hypericum to help heal cuts. Peppermint leaves made into a tea are helpful for trapped wind and referred pain. Once your scar has begun to heal, then vitamin E cream can help reduce its appearance.

Once you are home, get as much rest as possible, drink lots of water to flush out your system and be sure not to lift anything heavier than your baby. That means very few household chores (phew!), no vacuuming and other strenuous tasks but also no lifting a toddler if you have one of those. If your little one needs a bit of love, offer a cuddle rather than a carry, and place a pillow over your scar to shield you from any potentially painful prods with little knees and elbows.

Doing simple physiotherapy exercises in the early days is a good idea – deep breathing into the chest, and simple circling your ankles in bed – to keep your circulation going, but wait until after your postnatal check-up before doing anything more strenuous. One thing every new mother should be doing is her pelvic floor exercises (see page 167). While there are entire cultures of women who opt for Caesareans in an attempt to 'conserve' their pelvic floor, the truth is that the weight of the pregnant uterus will have put the muscles under pressure anyway and so pelvic floor exercises are still essential to protect you against incontinence.

Birth After Caesareans

One of the most common questions a mother asks after having a Caesarean is 'Will I have another Caesarean next time around?' Some women ask because they want to be able to have one – once you have had a Caesarean, it seems easier to find grounds for having a second one. If you have had a difficult labour that ended in a Caesarean, then it is completely understandable that you'd like to be a little bit more prepared second or third time around. More often, though, women ask the question because they still feel, even after a good Caesarean experience, that they would like the chance to have a natural birth. It is not uncommon for women, despite the highest levels of care and even when there was no alternative to having a Caesarean, to still feel robbed of their birth experience and want the chance to give birth naturally. In my experience, no amount of me telling a woman that it was necessary, and she should in no way feel like a failure, takes from the fact that for some – possibly deep-rooted reason – many women feel an urge to do it the way nature intended. Don't get me wrong – some women are emboldened and empowered by their Caesareans, but many are also left feeling a little disheartened.

There is a now century-old and somewhat notorious quote, 'Once a Caesarean, always a Caesarean,' uttered by a Dr Edward Cragin, which was, for a long time, the standard answer to the 'Will I have another Caesarean?' question (and in some places the old adage is still a gospel). But in the UK, VBAC (vaginal birth after Caesarean) is now increasingly common. The worry used to be that the Caesarean scar might rupture when a woman went into labour with another child, but since the advent of the transverse incision, which heals as a much stronger scar, the rupture risk is small (0.35 per cent according to the NICE guidelines on Caesareans, though this increases dramatically with an induction). Despite this, and the mountains of research that support the validity and benefits of natural births after Caesareans, there are some obstetricians who are still uncomfortable with what is often referred to as a 'trial of labour' and who feel the need to scare women out of it as an option without giving them the true picture.

And this is despite the fact that the VBAC success rate is very high – about three-quarters of women who opt for a VBAC manage to have a natural birth instead of a Caesarean next time around. What's more, those women are all the happier for it. While not everyone professes to have a 'dreamy' natural birth, a huge proportion proclaim it as having been a really positive experience: healing, empowering and emboldening.

'I was determined,' said a second-time mother from North London, 'to have a natural birth second time around. And I have to confess I felt amazing afterwards. In fact, I am sure having had the Caesarean first time made the experience of natural birth even more of an achievement for me. I felt like I had really conquered something.'

If you think you might want to try for a natural birth after having had one or even two Caesareans, then make sure you prepare yourself. In many cases you will be actively encouraged to go for a natural birth, but in others you might well have to be clever – find out all you can about VBACs, arm yourself with knowledge as well as confidence, be willing to shop around for care, and stay open-minded (as well as determined, if necessary) throughout. There are several organisations that would be more than willing to help if you come up against resistance – AIMS (see page 268) being probably the best first port of call.

There are as many different birth experiences as there are babies, and the positive experience/negative experience line is not drawn by the mode of birth. For every woman who has had a difficult natural birth, there is another for whom the experience was amazing. And the world of Caesareans is the same. For some it is the pinnacle of their life, every bit as amazing as the natural version, while others feel downbeat about it. Being empowered and at the centre of your own experience, natural or otherwise, is more often the deal-breaker for a woman. So whether you are faced with your first Caesarean or a VBAC, arm yourself with information and be positive. It might sound a little happy-clappy, but the truth is, just like with natural birth, mindset is everything.

SUMMARY

- The World Health Organization says only 10 to 15 per cent of women should need any intervention in their births.

- For those women, a Caesarean can be a fantastic safety net and we should be grateful for the operation.

- There are certain unequivocal reasons for a Caesarean and if you are faced with the inevitable, then try to see it as a positive.

- Obviously it is harder to influence your experience when you have a Caesarean, but there are still ways to personalise it – for example, asking for your partner to announce the baby's sex, requesting to see your baby born and having skin-to-skin contact immediately after the birth.

- If you know you have to have a Caesarean, and even if you don't, having an idea of the procedure will help on the day if your birth doesn't go according to plan.

- There are many women for whom a Caesarean birth is every bit as amazing as the natural version. Whatever happens, try to stay positive.

- Recovery from a Caesarean is slower than after a natural birth. Respect that you have had major abdominal surgery and get as much help in the early days and weeks as you can.

PART 3
Beyond the Birth

CHAPTER 9

The Babymoon
Saying No to Supermum

'I have found a kind of peace with you, especially when I am feeding. You have forced me to be still, to distil my life. I have shed all that is extraneous because, simply, there is no time any more for so much.'

Nikki Gemmell, *Tales of the Recent Past*

In many cultures all over the world there is a well-established tradition of what is often referred to as the 'babymoon' – a period straight after the birth of quiet adjustment to motherhood, quite unlike normal life. Usually the mother is doted on, physically and emotionally nurtured and relieved of all responsibility so that she can focus entirely on the adjustment to becoming a new mother and spending time with her newborn baby. In Colombia the new mother becomes the complete centre of attention for six weeks. She does not lift a finger, and nor is she expected to. In India, it is 21 days before a mother emerges with her baby to rejoin the community, having been secluded in a separate house, her needs met by a willing band of older women. When I got up after two weeks (which by modern standards borders on seriously lazy), my Brazilian friend was horrified: 'Go back to bed,' she almost yelled at me, tutting and shaking her head. 'You are a new mother. We should be looking after you.' In Brazil, women have the luxury of a three-week 'lying-in' period.

The New Modern Mother

This is all in sharp contrast to the modern Western woman's postnatal experience. Because of staff shortages postnatal care in most hospitals has been left desperately wanting for some time (unless you are privileged enough to pay for it), and now it is almost non-existent. Many of the large UK hospitals have a policy of discharging a woman after as little as four hours after the birth, and sometimes even before their baby has had the first feed. Long gone are the days when women could convalesce – even the word now sounds old-fashioned – for 10 days, when they were brought endless cups of tea, helped with feeding and guided as to how to nurture their baby. Now, a night in hospital is considered something of a luxury and more often than not needs to be bargained for. While many women say they are happy to get back to the comfort of their own home, once they are there it is often assumed that life is back to normal. Yet nothing could be further from the truth. There is nothing normal about the first few weeks of motherhood, not even second, third or fourth time around.

Physical Transformations

Physically, your body is going through a major transformation. Obviously the act of giving birth has taken you from being pregnant to not pregnant in one seemingly almighty bang, but the real metamorphosis takes much longer than that (and some women lament that they – or at least their stomachs – are never the same again!)

Over the first week your uterus will retract to its original size, which means going from something the size of a watermelon (and some) to something the size of a grapefruit. This process can actually be quite painful as it involves 'after pains' or small contractions. It is often the case that the quicker your birth, the more dramatic the after pains, and certainly they are worse after every child. It is common for you to feel them as you breastfeed – the oxytocin produced when you feed induces a small contraction of the uterus. Some women barely notice them, and they usually stop after a couple of days. In fact, all the body's organs that have been pushed and skewed by the growing baby and placenta, will take a little time to return to their rightful place, though most of this happens unbeknownst to mum who quite frankly has enough on her plate as it is.

It is also completely normal to feel like you are peeing almost constantly in the first few days after birth, as the body is ridding itself of the extra fluid that accumulates during pregnancy – anything from 2 to 8 litres!

Rather annoyingly for some mothers, the more noticeable external changes take much longer to return to normal. It is usual (and a bit depressing!) to still look pregnant even weeks after you have given birth. The stomach, which inevitably has had to stretch to accommodate the baby, can't just snap back like a bit of elastic (if only!) But rest assured it will slowly return to a version of normal over the weeks and months that follow. My advice is to wear your maternity clothes, but also go and treat yourself to some super-cheap, floaty dresses so that at least mentally you can distinguish between pre- and post-birth. Either that, or borrow something from a friend. Heaving yourself back into your huge maternity trousers when you are covered in baby sick and have bags under your eyes is going to do nothing for your state of mind. A pretty, if oversized, dress might just help.

I have to confess, I would be lying if I tried to pretend that the postnatal period wasn't a) at times difficult and b) fairly unglamorous. That doesn't mean it doesn't have its amazing moments – of course it does – but the harder stuff is there too, and all too often birth preparation books don't say very much about this time. If these publications are scared of putting mothers off having a baby, it's surely a bit late! We can safely assume that the vast majority of women reading a book on birth are already pregnant. There is a host of things that mothers can be faced with – apart from their newborn – which are common enough to warrant a mention.

We've talked about after pains. It is also normal to bleed after birth – known as 'lochia', this is the result of the womb shedding its lining. During the first week the bleeding will in all likelihood be quite heavy, and there can even be small clots of blood that pass through. Gradually, the bleeding tails off over the next few weeks, first becoming like a normal period and gradually easing, but it is likely to last up to a month. This will happen whether you have had a vaginal delivery or a Caesarean. If you have what seems to be crazily heavy bleeding, pain or any exceptionally large clots, then it is best to call your midwife – in the case of very heavy bleeding, call her immediately. If you have passed a very large clot, then try to keep the clot in the pad (uurgh, I know!) to show the midwife.

You may suffer from temporary incontinence after childbirth, which means you can find yourself leaking or, even worse, actually peeing yourself. In fact, I remember a girlfriend and I laughing hysterically – and almost peeing ourselves in the process – as we confessed to the inevitable 'peeing' ourselves after a long bath. This whole area is a lot less toned than it once was, and therefore water can go in when it shouldn't, and come out when it shouldn't! And sadly, a Caesarean doesn't protect you from this particular little pleasure – my hysterical friend had had one. It is imperative that you start your pelvic floor exercises (see page 167) as soon as you think of them, and that you do them religiously. Use the post-it note reminder on page 167 and follow the exercises in the same way. Even if you are not peeing yourself, you'll need to do them to prevent incontinence as you get older, and it can also seriously enhance your sex life (this will be the last thing on your mind in the early days, I know, but one day you will care, I promise).

Another common postnatal complaint is constipation. It usually happens in the first few days after birth and is the result of rapid hormone changes. Although eating a high-fibre diet might be the last thing on your mind, try to eat as much as you can – it is easy to include at breakfast if you buy a good-quality muesli or have high-fibre toast. Prune juice or some over-the-counter medicines, such as Lactulose or Fybogel, can also help, as will drinking loads and loads of water.

The other 'bottom' issue you can be faced with is 'piles'. I know, I also thought that only old people got piles, but I cannot tell you the number of postnatal mums who whisper in my ear that they have it. So if you do, don't be afraid to tell your midwife. In fact, while I don't want to create a generation of hypochondriacs, in the period straight after the birth I think it is worth mentioning anything that seems unusual to your midwife. After all, how are you supposed to know what might or might not happen?

Piles or haemorrhoids are basically varicose veins on or just inside the anus, which can be red or purple – they will sometimes bleed and can be very sore. Witch hazel ointment dabbed on with a small piece of cotton wool can help, as can placing some sanitary pads in the freezer and then using them when they are cold. There are also a number of over-the-counter remedies that can help – a good pharmacist will be able to advise you, as will your midwife.

The Emotional Bits

As well as these countless and decidedly unglamorous physical changes, one of the most trying parts of the postnatal period is the emotional upheaval. Not only have you become a mother, which although wonderful can simultaneously feel like you've been hit round the head with a cricket bat, but your hormones are all over the place, which means that you feel as though you are on one huge emotional roller-coaster ride. One day you are all doe-eyed, happy and infatuated with your little gorgeous milky-smelling bundle, and the next day you feel like a snivelling wreck, constantly crying and overwhelmed with the responsibility of it all. While this is hard, it is also completely and utterly normal. Rest assured that you are going through what the vast majority of other mothers go through. It might not mean much to you now, but on the blue days it is reassuring to know you are not alone (or strange, or ungrateful, or a bad mother).

The first, and probably most common, of these emotional surges happens about three or four days after the baby is born, and is aptly known as 'fourth day baby blues'. After the initial elation of having given birth to this amazing little package, your progesterone levels take a nose dive to make way for your 'milk' hormones, and in response you feel sad and weepy and as if you'd like to curl up in a little ball under the duvet all day and be intravenously fed tea. But, instead, there is a baby to deal with and probably an unsuspecting partner who hasn't read about this, or your own mother who has long forgotten her own experience. Fourth day baby blues is normal, and be reassured that it goes away. And there is not a lot you can do about it apart from close the front door, curl up in bed, arm yourself with a steady supply of tissues and distract yourself with a really good romcom or even a tearjerker. At least then you have a focus for your tears. The homeopathic remedy Pulsatilla can also help – take a single 200c dose. Strip your diary back, cancel things if necessary and lay low.

Have a good cry, if needs be, and call a friend who has been there before and so understands. In fact, anyone who has ever been a mother will understand.

The other tricky bit about the first few weeks is that the baby has very little rhythm to her nights and days. As a result, it is very easy to get caught up in the idea that this is what life will be like for evermore. Yet rhythms establish themselves slowly, and trying to force a baby into a strict schedule right from the beginning is often futile. Your baby is also adjusting to something wholly new – seeing light, breathing through her lungs and digesting for the first time. Her sense of night and day and that sleep follows a bath or that food follows sleep will develop slowly. Try not to be in a rush. You can nudge your baby into a semblance of day and night at this stage, but trying too hard or being too rigid will just frustrate you. Rest assured, if it's a rhythm you want then you will be able to develop one slowly. You will also eventually get your evenings back to yourself. It all takes time, but as my father-in-law said to me after the birth of my second child, 'It is not a marathon. You are not trying to get anywhere.' Whatever you do, take it slowly at the beginning. If you do, it is actually even possible to enjoy these early weeks. You are two people getting to know each other for the first time, and the more you allow that to happen slowly and gently the more you will enjoy it. Second-time mothers always seem to take more time, and worry less about what they might be missing out on – and they all say it's because they realise how quickly it goes and how precious that time can be. In a world where life is eternally busy and we spend so much of it running from one thing to another, the excuse to do nothing but what is essential can be a blessing if you choose to see it that way.

Coping With It All

All too often women say that they felt (more or less) prepared for the birth, but wholly unprepared for everything that comes after. 'No one told me it was going to be so hard' is an all too common cry amongst postnatal groups. And while women very often talk about how amazing they felt after giving birth, and how precious those weeks are with a little baby, these positive emotions are often bound up with many others – a sense of being overwhelmed, a genuine fear that they don't know how to mother, exhaustion or difficulties breastfeeding. While it seems easy nowadays to prepare for the birth if you choose to, it is still very difficult to truly prepare for the period afterwards. Motherhood is something that we seem to learn on the hoof, but there are some things you can do to make the period a little easier, both physically and emotionally. The list that follows is a practical guide to what you might need – having all of these things to hand means you will have less to think about once your baby has arrived.

The Babymoon Shopping List

FOR YOU

Sanitary pads – lots of thick ones for the early days and then some thinner ones for the weeks that follow. Don't at this stage use a tampon.

A plastic measuring jug – it can sting to pee the first couple of days after birth, even if you haven't torn or had stitches. Try to do your first pee in the bath or shower, but after that have a plastic jug next to the loo, and before you go, fill it with warm water and pour it on yourself as you pee. This completely takes away the stinging sensation.

Nipple cream – try the one sold by the Active Birth Centre (see page 268), or some health food stores now stock papaya ointment from Australia, which is completely fantastic. So much so that if you can't find it in the UK, but have an Australian friend, it would be worth getting them to send some over. Otherwise pure lanolin also works very well.

Thank-you cards and stamps – you will in all likelihood get oodles of flowers and presents in the first few days and weeks (maybe slightly fewer if it's your second baby and even less if it's your third, and I imagine by your fourth you can not bother with this bit!) Having cards and stamps beside the bed means you can write your thank yous and pass them to your partner to post on his way out the door. A lot of baby books say don't bother with thank yous, but for those of you who like the ritual, having everything to hand makes it much easier.

A flask and herbal tea bags – no matter what routine you eventually do or don't get your baby into, at first there will be night-time feeds. I found it really useful to keep the lights down low, turn on the radio (volume low) and make myself a cup of herbal tea as I settled down to feed my babies. It meant that at the beginning at least, I didn't mind getting up so much. In fact, dare I confess it, I now occasionally hear the shipping forecast and it brings back rather lovely (possibly rose-tinted) memories of the smell of newborns and little fingers and toes! And, on a practical level, a herbal tea such as fennel or peppermint will help you get back to sleep (as if you need help!) It was also the ingenious idea of a friend of mine to have a flask of hot water by the bed, boiled before you hunker down, to save you from switching on the kettle in the middle of the night. If you don't like herbal teas, don't substitute it with a caffeine-filled alternative. Maybe try a Horlicks?

At least two, possibly three, sets of pyjamas – they are better than nighties as you can unbutton the top or lift it up to feed, rather than hoist up your entire nightie (and if it's winter, freeze your socks off in the process!)

Homeopathic remedies – Arnica and Bellis Perennis for bruising or, if you have it, use the Helios birth kit. It is as good postnatally as it is for the birth. I highly recommend it as an investment.

Breast pads – you'll need them, trust me. And they won't stop you smelling of coagulated milk most of the time, even if you change them regularly, which you'll need to. A little plastic bag by the bed is also really useful for soaked breast pads. You can either get several sets of washable pads (in which case get more than you think you'll need – they seem to be like socks and get lost in the washing machine) or disposable ones (much more practical but obviously much less 'green').

Maternity bras – in a larger than expected size, usually!

A feel-good, easy-to-read book – if you are on your second or third baby, you might not have time. But first time round it means you will stay seated or lying down for more of the day, which is what you should be doing.

Water bottle – regularly filled up by your partner or anyone else who is around and helping out. You will get unbelievably thirsty when you breastfeed, so you must drink a lot more water than you think. It also helps to avoid constipation (see page 203), which is common after birth.

Paracetamol – in case your after pains (see page 201) really hurt, which they can, especially if it is your second or third baby. There are also some good homeopathic remedies for after pains – Secale 200c if you've had lots of children or the pain is long lasting, Cimicifuga 200c if the pain is concentrated in the groin area and is quite intense, and Arnica 200c if it's worse when the baby feeds – which it very often is.

A hot-water bottle – not for any particular purpose except that it feels nurturing and cosy, especially if your baby is a winter one. It can also help with after pains if you are suffering unduly from those.

Toys, puzzles and colouring books with crayons – these are not for you (pregnancy has not made you regress that much!), but on the list for second- or third-time mums, who might have an older child who wants some attention. I found it really good to be able to do puzzles with one hand while feeding the baby with the other, and if they are close to hand you have an instant fix for a possibly put-out older child.

Frozen food – one good way of satisfying your nesting instinct and preparing in advance is cooking and freezing loads of lovely nutritious meals And don't worry about having the odd ready meals; served with a bit of broccoli or some other vegetable or salad on the side they will keep you well fed quickly and with minimal mess.

In addition to the above it might be useful to have:

Contact details for a breastfeeding counsellor (have it by the bed and at the first sign of trouble feeding or latching on, call her) or the nearest breastfeeding clinic – this support is worth its weight in gold. By getting the contact details in advance, you'll know who to call. And while you are compiling a list, put your best friend's and your midwife's number on there as well – in case you need a good laugh or cry (and you'll probably need both at some point) or you have anything that you are worried about.

FOR THE BABY

Newborn babies need surprisingly little, which is not what a trip to your local department store or Mothercare would suggest. Gadgets, play mats, fandangle pushchairs and the like are all well and good but you don't need nearly as much as you think.

But you do need *lots of little babygros*. Try to borrow as many as possible, or buy them second-hand as your baby will grow out of them *so* quickly. It is not unusual for newborns to get through six or so a day, with their exploding nappies and sick and dribble (all sounds lovely, doesn't it?!) Don't get babygros with poppers at the back, or too many poppers for that matter, as it makes it infinitely more difficult to change your baby, which you are obviously going to be doing quite often. And if you'll excuse my little sales pitch – if you can get your hands on any stretchy Bonds Babygros from Australia, then buy a truck-load. They are the king of babygros!

A sling – when you have had your week in bed or on the sofa, you might want to venture out into the big wide world. A sling for the first trip is a really good idea. Remember, it might feel strange to you to see that the world hasn't stopped since you've given birth and gone underground, but the first experience of the outside will be infinitely stranger for your little one, who will be experiencing outside light and sounds and cold air for the first time. A sling is a much cosier, more protected place to be than a pushchair.

Lots of newborn nappies, cotton wool and a little bowl for warm water – this is best to use for changing nappies in the early days and you can, if you want to, progress on to unscented baby wipes eventually as they are much easier to use. Remember, however, that a newborn baby's skin is quite sensitive so to begin with they can cause a rash.

Lots of skin-to-skin contact and hugs – this is added on as a seeming jovial postscript but it is absolutely not to be trivialised. Babies thrive on contact – in fact they actively need it – and the more you can hold a baby at the beginning the happier and more settled she will be. In fact, nature is incredible; there is actually a system called thermal synchrony whereby if a baby is lying on her mother's chest and is cold, then the mother's body temperature will increase to warm the baby up, and likewise, if a baby's temperature rises too much, the mother's will fall in accordance. It is why 'kangaroo care', which is a way of nurturing premature babies by strapping them to their mother, skin-to-skin, is as successful in many cases as an incubator and sometimes more so.

As well as all these little practicalities, there are other things to consider which might help you enjoy rather than wish away the first few weeks and months.

Allow Yourself a Babymoon

To start, heed the advice of a wonderful midwife by the name of Annie Francis who advises 'one week in bed and one week on the sofa'. If you decide in advance that you are going to allow yourself that luxury, you will already be in a mindset that accepts that life will not go immediately back to normal and you'll behave accordingly. Don't make plans for the immediate postnatal period and when you do start venturing out, plan one thing at a time. In the early weeks, limit visitors. It is tempting to agree to a visit from every aunt, uncle, cousin and friend who wants to wet the baby's head, but conjuring up the energy to be sparky and vibrant can be exhausting. If you don't feel like it, don't do it. For the first week at least, stay in pyjamas or floppy 'I am not going anywhere' clothes. That way, you won't be inclined to do too much, and if people come to see you, it is clear that they should be getting you the cups of tea and not the other way round. The absolute best guests we ever had after the birth of our second child were friends who came over, made us laugh, made the tea and left after an hour or so, leaving a particularly delicious kedgeree in the kitchen ready for us to eat that night. We had company, good chat and supper made for us all in one fell swoop!

SLEEP WHEN YOUR BABY SLEEPS

The next thing is something you will be told 1,000 times and I can almost guarantee that you probably won't do it. Or if you do, it won't be enough. It is the advice to 'sleep when the baby sleeps'. For as long as your baby is not entirely sure of the distinction between day and night, and while her tummy is the size of a 1p coin, you will be getting broken sleep during the night, to a greater or lesser degree, depending on the baby and your parenting rituals, but broken nonetheless. To save yourself from the insanity that comes from sleep deprivation, you need to try to catch up on sleep whenever you can. Easier said than done, I know, when there is laundry to do, meals to cook, a house that looks like a bomb has hit it and a needy toddler who wants your attention. But, if it is at all possible, take power naps. Even those little micro-sleeps – the shortest possible version of a power nap – can help. And if it is a choice between doing a load of washing or having a nap, have the nap first. The washing can go on when the baby has been fed and is happily gurgling in her Moses basket or snuggled against you in a sling. It is absolutely true that you will not regret having had a nap, and will never feel as though you are sleeping too much. Sleep might feel like an indulgence but it is not – it's a necessity. There is a strong belief that postnatal depression is in part brought on by lack of sleep.

ACCEPT HELP

Try not to think of paternity leave as the same as a holiday. While it is tempting to take advantage of your partner being around to do lovely things together, especially as a newly formed, or newly changed family, the point of him being at home is to look after you and the baby. Allow yourself to be looked after – breakfast, lunch and dinner in bed if needs be – and, as well as your partner (if he is about), enlist the help of absolutely everyone who offers – mothers, mothers-in-law, sisters and friends. Remember that eventually paternity leave ends, and all the offers of help gradually dry up. If you are one of those stoic, I can do it women (and too many of us are), try to put that attitude to one side for a bit and enjoy being looked after. Eventually you will be on your own, and will long for the opportunity you once had to get an extra bit of shut-eye while granny took the baby for a walk, or the indulgence of a long bath in the afternoon while daddy was around to gurgle at the little one. And if you can't face doing it for yourself, do it for everyone else. They will be itching to get to know and bond with the baby, so allowing everyone a bit of quality time is a good thing all around.

Finally, allow yourself, if at all possible, the odd indulgence. If you are off to have a long soak in a bath, then really go to town; fill it with lovely aromatherapy oils or some luxurious bubbles, light a scented candle and settle down with a magazine (and an assurance that the hot water is on for a top-up). These little luxuries have an exaggerated significance in the weeks after the birth. And in my opinion they are not luxuries at all, but absolute necessities.

SUMMARY

- The days and weeks immediately after your baby is born are a special, and very unusual, time.
- You are going through huge emotional and physical changes, as well as adjusting to the whole idea that you are now responsible for this very new little person.
- Getting back to normal will be very low down on your list of priorities.
- Give yourself as much time as you need and strip your diary right back. Remember, you are not trying to get anywhere and should have nothing to do.
- Accept as much help as possible, even if it is not something you are used to doing. You wont regret it.

- Get as much sleep as you can – the power nap version if necessary. You are recovering from the birth and your body is undergoing a massive transformation to return to its pre-pregnant state.

- Don't fret about getting your baby into a rhythm or routine straight away. She, too, is adjusting to everything and will gradually settle as the days and weeks go by.

- If you have days when you feel down or overwhelmed, then remember that it is normal, and try to talk to someone – your partner, a good friend, your own mother or your midwife. Every new mother has great highs as well as difficult lows.

- Allow yourself the odd indulgence – a long, lazy bath, a breakfast out, a new pair of shoes – goodness knows, you of all people deserve it!

skip this chapter.
Usual Bullshit.

CHAPTER 10

Breastfeeding
Beyond the Slogans

'Breastfeeding problems are greatest in societies where everyone wears a watch and least in societies where no one wears a watch.'
Jack Newman

'Feed like a gypsy. Take no notice of the clock.'
Grandmother Wisdom

'Breast is Best', 'The Feed-good Factor', 'You can't get fitter than a breastfed nipper'. Wherever you look, breastfeeding slogans abound. Internet sites are awash with complaints by mothers who feel the message is pushed on them and with stories of mothers who feel guilty if they can't feed in the face of this apparent 'pressure'. Yet breastfeeding rates in the UK are the lowest in all of Europe. In 2005, only 35 per cent of babies were being exclusively breastfed, and that came down to 3 per cent at five months.[31] This is crazily low when compared to Sweden – where 98 per cent of mothers breastfeed their babies at the outset and 88 per cent continue to do so well after they are six months old.

....

The truth is, love or loathe them, the slogans just don't seem to be working.

We might all have heard the messages, but the truth is most of us probably don't really know what lies beneath them. And, more importantly, the modern mother is a very isolated beast, all too often hot-footed out the hospital door at the earliest opportunity, often with very little back-up and unarmed with the most basic skills. In a culture where breastfeeding happens largely behind closed doors, we need to be shown what to do, often more than once, and yet home alone there is often no one to do the demonstrating. Mothers often confess to me that they feel guilty for not breastfeeding, yet it is not the mother who is at fault. Their inability to feed has almost certainly got nothing to do with their physical make-up, and even less to do with their mental stamina. The truth is, we are simply not supported to breastfeed.

The good news is that cultural turnarounds are entirely possible. In Norway in 1970 only 20 per cent of mothers breastfed their babies, but now 99 per cent do.[32] There, as in most of the Scandinavian countries, it is considered the most normal and natural thing. And, unsurprisingly, women in those countries find it much easier than we do.

Why Bother to Breastfeed?

YOUR BABY'S HEALTH

The benefits of breastfeeding are many, and well documented. As much as the slogans might annoy you, they aren't lying. Though it is hard to distinguish how much of the benefit comes from the milk and how much from the particular kind of nurture a breast-fed baby gets, the pluses are too good to ignore. Breastfed babies tend to be healthier than their bottle-fed counterparts, with less incidence of ear infections, fewer allergies, less vomiting and diarrhoea, and less pneumonia, wheezing and bronchitis. Their long-term health is also boosted. Exclusive breastfeeding for four months can reduce the chances of some nasty childhood diseases such as diabetes, leukaemia, and liver and bowel disease. Of course, it is possible to find perfectly healthy bottle-fed babies, but if you can give your baby a leg-up in the health stakes, is it not worth a shot at least?

COMFORT

And there's more. As well as benefits to a baby's physical health, breastfeeding is also a great comfort to a newborn. The physical proximity to the mother, as well as the hours of touch that breast-feeding entails, and the daily dose of the love hormone oxytocin that gets transferred in the breast milk will make a baby feel more connected, more secure and altogether more calm.

HORMONE PICK-ME-UP

Rather wonderfully, it is not just the baby who benefits. What is much less talked about (goodness knows why) is quite how much breastfeeding is of benefit to you, too. Believe it or not, once any initial hurdles have been overcome, breastfeeding can actually make mothering easier.

Whenever you feed, you and the baby are given a dose of oxytocin, the rather wonderful love hormone that I have mentioned so often in this book. This is the same hormone that makes you feel good around a dinner table, and the very same one that makes you feel all dopey and loved up after an orgasm. It means that every time you feed, you are given a natural little pick-me-up, except that it is a calm-me-down, and it really helps you to bond with your baby.

As well as oxytocin, there is another little treasure that is produced in response to breastfeeding – prolactin. As well as being responsible for lactation, prolactin is also said to have an effect on your brain, making you infinitely more capable of dealing with the mundane. While I would never want to belittle mothering, I would be lying if I didn't say it involves a very healthy dose of the mundane. Repetition is a constant, and anything that helps us embrace it can only be a good thing. And as well as tolerance, prolactin enhances your resistance to stress, your maternal feelings and behaviour, and it acts as a natural analgesic. With all these beneficial hormones flooding your system on a daily basis, expect a bit of a slump in your mood when you eventually stop breastfeeding – many mothers recognise it, though few can explain what it is. It's an unfortunate process, in which you are adjusting to the demands of motherhood but now without any of the hormonal help.

EASE

A common complaint from modern mothers is that breastfeeding ties you down to your baby. While this is undeniable, it is possible to express milk to allow your partner or somebody else to help with the odd feed. And it is also true that being forced to be with your baby is not all bad. Many mothers say to me that with hindsight they relished the fact that they needed to strip their lives back a little and not try to do so much in the early months and weeks. When you are in the thick of early motherhood it is hard to see your way out, but there is absolutely no doubt that you will look back and marvel at how quickly it all went, and even miss those foggy days when it was just you and your very tiny baby. They are not babies for very long.

YOUR HEALTH

Health-wise, breastfeeding also brings benefits for you. It burns an extra 500 calories a day so, as long as you don't live by the adage 'eating for two', your chances of fitting back into your jeans and of being healthier in the process are increased. More importantly, breastfeeding reduces the risk of menopausal breast cancer, as well as ovarian cancer and of hip fracture later in life.

CONVENIENCE

What's more, it is incredibly convenient. Breast milk is always available, served up at exactly the right temperature, doesn't need all the clobber of sterilisers and bottles and is free (saving you a very nice £450 a year, thank you very much – that's a new dress, pair of boots and some).

With all of these undeniable benefits, the best possible advice anyone can give you is to try it – every single day of feeding is beneficial, so even if you don't continue with it as long as you might like, you will have chalked up a good dose of antibodies for your baby and a few quick fixes of oxytocin for yourself. It is worth, at least, a try.

So How Does it Work?

Rest assured, the chances are you will be able to feed your baby. Only about 1 per cent of women cannot. The size and shape of your breasts doesn't influence the amount of milk you produce so, big or small, you are capable of being part of a long line of women, 2,000 generations of mothers it works out as, who successfully breastfed before the advent of formula feed. Rather annoyingly, this long lineage doesn't make breastfeeding as instinctive as you might assume it to be. Babies seem to know exactly what to do, but we need a little more guidance. And this is especially so in the UK where it is not at all common to see women feeding in public and when you do, the magic technique is usually hidden under a shawl or a strategically placed bit of muslin. But we can all re-learn the art of breastfeeding, and with a little guidance and in some cases persistence, breastfeeding can soon feel like second nature.

AT THE BEGINNING

The best way to establish breastfeeding is to get babies feeding as soon as possible after birth. That does not have to mean immediately, and you certainly shouldn't rush or force the process, but the aim is to try to get them feeding within an hour of the birth, after which they usually fall into a deep sleep. If they haven't fed at the outset, then it can make feeding harder to establish later on. Begin by allowing your baby skin-to-skin contact with you and just wait patiently for the signs that she might want to feed. Babies are literally programmed to seek out their mother's milk, and as long as a baby has had a normal birth, she will begin to portray all the signs of a baby in search of the breast – nuzzling, an open mouth, and even wriggling towards the nipple. In fact, there is now a whole library of video footage (just YouTube 'baby crawl') of babies who nuzzle around and use their kicking reflex to seek out the breast and latch themselves on. If you've never seen the footage, I highly recommend you seek it out. It is completely fascinating and, if nothing else, it will give you faith in Mother Nature. The theory is that babies are attracted to the smell of the breast milk, which is like that of amniotic fluid, and that this, coupled with their instincts, guides them to the nipple. In fact, experiments were done where mothers had one breast washed and the other left as it was, and the babies always went towards the unwashed breast.[33] Along the same lines, an experiment was done where babies were placed next to fresh breast pads, and those that smelt of their mother's milk. Unsurprisingly, left to their own devices they all inched towards the milk-soaked pad.

Wait until the baby begins to show signs of interest in feeding. By all means, try to allow your baby to 'crawl' up and latch on if you'd like to, though often a midwife might equally want to gently help the process along, encouraging you to hold your baby at chest height, and trying to ensure that the baby gets a good mouthful of breast. As feeding for both mother and baby are so hormonally influenced, the conditions and your state of mind matter – it is important that in the first few hours, or even days, you are relaxed, and feel unobserved yet well supported. Privacy at this early stage is still very important.

For the first 24 hours a baby can feed very little – sometimes as little as two teaspoons – and will very often sleep a lot. In fact if I had a pound for every parent who has told me proudly that quite unexpectedly their baby slept through the night on their first night, I would be a very rich woman. I am always loath to burst their bubble and tell them that it is no indication of how they might sleep for the first year!

After the first day, your baby will tend to wake up a little more, and on day two or three will often feed seemingly constantly. In the early days she is feasting on a thick yellow substance called colostrum, which is both medical as well as nutritional. Colostrum is full to the brim of antibodies, and works also as a natural laxative, encouraging a baby to pass through their first poo. Meconium (as the first poo is called) is thick, black and very sticky, as you will discover when you try to wipe it off your baby's bottom – concrete is nothing by comparison. Incidentally, colostrum also contains sugar and protein for energy.

Colostrum is followed after a couple of days by a transitional milk, which is very rich and creamy, and then the more established or mature milk, which is a combination of thinner foremilk to quench thirst, and then fat-rich hindmilk to help the baby gain weight. What is quite extraordinary about your milk, and which cannot be matched by formula, is the way in which its composition changes according to the needs of your baby, her age and the time of day. It will even change in accordance with the weather, becoming more diluted and therefore more thirst quenching as the thermometer rises, which is why breastfed babies don't need water top-ups in hotter weather.

SUPPLY AND DEMAND

Breastfeeding works according to the laws of supply and demand, whereby the baby suckles and a message is sent to the mother's brain to produce milk, so the more suckling there is, the more milk is produced. This is why a baby naturally feeds non-stop a day or two after birth – by doing so she is encouraging your milk to 'come in'. By day three or four (sometimes a little later in mothers who have had a Caesarean) you'll have a dramatic drop in progesterone and a concurrent rise in prolactin, which brings on lactation or your 'proper' milk. With your milk coming on thick and fast, your breasts can also get engorged, which makes them feel hot, swollen and sore. Even if you are small-breasted, you are in all likelihood going to rival Dolly Parton for a day or two – and it's much less fun than you might ever have imagined! Rest assured it is only because your supply is exceeding demand and it will settle itself in a day or two. In the meantime there are a few things you can do to relieve the pressure and therefore the discomfort. Contrary to what a lot of people tell you, it is absolutely fine to express a little bit of milk, and it is well worth doing. It will reduce the sheer amount in your breasts, but it also enables your baby to feed with a good mouthful of breast. If you need to take gentle pain relief, then by all means do – paracetamol or ibuprofen is a good idea (just avoid aspirin as it is not compatible with breast-feeding). There is also something of an old wives' tale, though Australians in particular swear by it, which is to place a cold, uncooked cabbage leaf in your bra. This is meant to reduce engorgement, though I have to confess that all it did for me was make me smell of humid cabbage – another reason for tears! But by all means try it and see how it works for you. Some people swear it makes a difference.

LATCHING ON

At the beginning your only focus should be on getting a good 'latch', which is a good attachment between the baby's mouth and your breast. Its success depends on the two of you, mother and baby, being in the right position. As most breastfeeding problems can be traced back to a poor latch, cracking this at the beginning is absolutely key.

When a baby has a good mouthful of breast (or more specifically areola), the nipple is effectively bypassed. This means the nipple doesn't get sore from being sucked on, and the milk ducts – which lie in the fatty tissue of the breast – get well stimulated so that the milk production and flow is good.

While I would highly recommend books that show you how to latch on, DVDs are even better. Even better, get a midwife to show you first, and then get her to watch you every time you latch on for the first few feeds, just to check that you are getting it right. If at any point you feel you have problems, then go to a breastfeeding clinic to get some advice from a lactation consultant. They are trained in the art of breastfeeding, and will have consistent and sound advice. It is persistence and crucially support at this stage that will make the difference between a good and bad experience. Have the telephone number of a recommended lactation consultant by your bed, so if you are at all worried you don't need to waste time or energy trying to find one. Difficulties, if you have them, can be really emotionally wearing, so you will never regret making things as easy as possible for yourself in advance. Thankfully, while wearing, problems are also easily rectified with the right help, which is essential to remember when you are in the thick of it. Whatever you do, do not be afraid to ask for help.

If your baby is latched on well, her sucking will stimulate the nerve endings in the breast, which then transmit a message to your pituitary gland (or 'back brain', just like during the birth), which releases the relevant hormones: prolactin, which produces the milk, and oxytocin, which stimulates the let-down reflex. This reflex actually contracts the little muscles around the glands in the breast, which squeezes the milk into ducts and then down to the nipple. The let-down reflex can feel a little strange at first, especially in the early days and weeks of feeding, and is like a buzzing or tingling sensation in the breasts. If you don't feel the let-down reflex, then don't be alarmed – some women never do. And in the vast majority it will take until day 10 or 12 before you feel anything at all. Be assured that so long as your baby is latched on well, she will be getting what she needs whether you feel the let-down reflex or not.

ARE YOU SITTING COMFORTABLY?

To begin with, get comfortable. Sit as upright as you can, supported by cushions behind your lower back, and have your feet flat on the floor (or on a pile of books if they don't reach). This is a good position in the early days of breastfeeding; once you have been feeding successfully for several weeks, you can be a lot more relaxed about your position, as long as the baby is still latched on properly. But being quite pedantic in the beginning will pay dividends in the long run.

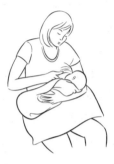

If this is your second or even third baby, try to go back to basics at the beginning. The way you feed an older baby or toddler, which will have been your last breastfeeding experience, is very different to feeding a newborn.

Make sure that the room is quiet and that you feel calm. It is a good idea to have a glass of water within reach, as breastfeeding makes you unbelievably thirsty.

Hold your baby with her belly to your chest and her head part way down your arm – if she is in the crook of your elbow, she is too far up and will be approaching the nipple from above. You want her approaching from slightly below the nipple. If you want to hold your baby to direct her, gently support her at the back of the neck or the base of her head rather than holding the whole of her head – you want to allow her the freedom of movement to flex her head back. Make sure her body is aligned – you should be able to draw a straight line from the top of her head, all the way down her spine to her tailbone.

Wait for your baby to open her mouth as wide as possible, as though she is yawning, and then bring the baby to the breast, her nose to your nipple. Don't lean forward or bring your breast to the baby as it will be uncomfortable for you, and will be the wrong angle for your baby.

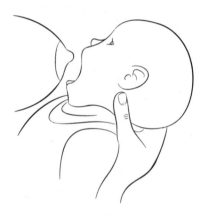

If the angle is right, your baby's nose will be at the nipple and she will have taken a big mouthful of breast that includes all or most of the areola. Her chin should be tucked into the breast, and her nose free to breathe. If you can see some of the areola, then it should be above not below the nipple. With her head tilted in this way the nipple will be drawn back, bypassing the tongue and positioned at the back of the baby's mouth.

Once your baby is latched on, and so long as you are relatively calm and relaxed, her sucking will stimulate the tingly let-down reflex. If it takes some time, just breathe out, relax your shoulders and wait patiently. It will happen. If your let-down is fast, your baby might gulp for a few moments as the milk is literallly squirted into her mouth, before settling into a gentle, comfortable rhythm.

SIGNS THAT THE BABY IS LATCHED ON CORRECTLY

- Her lower lip is rolled back, as though she is pouting.
- After an initial few gulps, she should settle into a slow, rhythmical sucking.
- The sucking should be evident at the jaw, rather than in the cheeks (so it is not the sort of sucking you do on a straw).
- Your nipple should be distended when you finish the feed, but not compressed.
- You should feel a tugging on the nipple, but not any sharp pain.
- Your breasts should feel emptied after a feed (though in the very early days, before the supply/demand balance has been sorted out, you might feel very little difference).
- Your baby's nose should be free for her to breathe through.
- Your baby should get satisfied by the feed, and stop suckling of her own accord.

If the latch is not right, then don't just pull your baby off the nipple – this will make your nipples sore. Break the suction by placing your little finger in the side of your baby's mouth, and then take her off. Readjust your own position, and that of the baby's, and then try again.

OTHER POSITIONS

Feeding your baby in the traditional tummy to breast way is not the only option and, as you get more experienced, you might want to try a variety of positions. My advice would be to crack one position first so that when you try out other ways, you know you have something easy and comfortable to fall back on.

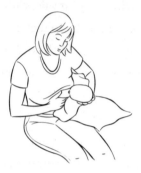

The rugby hold is a position that is commonly used if a baby expresses a preference for one breast, which they often do. By using the rugby hold on one side, you can 'trick' the baby into thinking it is the breast she likes. It often works. The 'rugby' hold is aptly named, as it involves tucking the baby up under your arm like a rugby ball, so her body is wrapped around the side of your body. Her head should still be level with your breast, and positioned nose to nipple, big mouthful of breast, chin tucked into the breast and nose free to breathe. Use cushions to support both you and your baby if necessary, and certainly in the beginning.

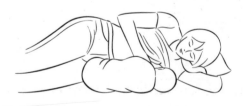

It is also possible to feed while lying down and Caesarean mothers are often taught this technique so that they can feed and avoid undue pressure on their scar. Again, the same basic principles apply, but this time you are lying on your side, with your head flat or very slightly raised. Position your baby, so that her head is slightly below the breast, with her nose in line with your nipple. Again, her body should be in a straight line, from head to spine to bottom.

HOW MUCH, HOW OFTEN?

The best advice for a new mother is to breastfeed 'little and often'. When a baby is born, her tummy is only the size of a 1p coin, which means she can only hold about 5–7 ml of milk in her tummy at any one time. By day three her tummy has grown to something the size of a ping-pong ball and by day 10, it's like a large chicken egg. Breast milk is easily digested, which is one of its benefits, hence the 'little and often' approach.

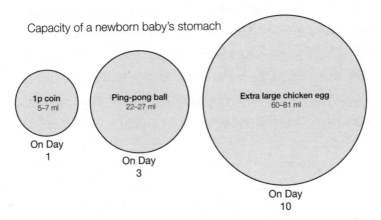

Capacity of a newborn baby's stomach

1p coin
5–7 ml

On Day 1

Ping-pong ball
22–27 ml

On Day 3

Extra large chicken egg
60–81 ml

On Day 10

In the early stages, trying to find a rhythm or routine is futile. It is best, during the first few weeks at least, to feed on demand

and allow the supply and demand balance to settle gently. Try also to stick just to breastfeeding at this stage as any topping up, or a kindly nurse bottle-feeding in the night, will influence your supply and interrupt the whole balancing act. You want your boobs to take their cue from your baby. Remember, there is no rush – you can use the coming weeks to gently nudge your baby into a rhythm if that is what you'd like, but at this stage you are just both getting started. Establishing breastfeeding takes time, patience and dedication, so clear the decks and try to get as much help as possible around the house, so that you can curl up and focus exclusively on your new baby, feeding as often as necessary.

Begin by offering one breast, and allow your baby to drain that one completely. This will ensure she gets her share of both the thirst-quenching foremilk and the fatty, hunger-satisfying hindmilk, which will ensure she gains the weight she needs. You can then offer up the other breast. At the beginning, she might not want it – it won't take much to fill that little tummy, but as she grows she will take more and more milk during each feed. (The duration of each feed will actually reduce as you both become better at the feeding process.) When you come to the next feed, start with the breast you finished with last time. This can sometimes be very difficult to remember, especially as you are bound to be suffering from foggy baby brain, but you can use a bracelet or a brooch that you swap at each feed to remind you where you left off. You'll know you've reached the heady ranks of the experienced mother when you find yourself absent-mindedly handling your boobs to test which one is full or not!

Gradually your baby will begin to settle into a pattern, and over the coming weeks and months you can start to schedule your life around feeds, and even nudge your baby into something of a rhythm. Try to remain flexible, though, as rigid routines ignore the growth spurts that happen, on average, every six weeks or so – at these times it is not uncommon for a baby to feed almost non-stop for 24 hours. Many mothers unknowingly take this as a sign that they suddenly have insufficient milk, but it is not the case. The baby is sucking constantly to change the composition of the milk so that it accommodates her increasing need for fat. On these days, follow your baby's cues, cancel your plans and curl up on the sofa with countless cups of tea (fennel is great for milk production) and a good audio book.

For those of you who feel uncomfortable with no timing guidance at all, a general rule is that a one-week-old baby needs approximately 8–12 feeds in any 24-hour period, with a gap no longer than three hours between feeds. As the baby gets older, you can nudge her into a rhythm that distinguishes more between day and night. A good way to do that is to try to cluster feed in the evening, and then begin to establish an evening routine, perhaps of a bath and a feed and some gentle music, before putting your baby down to sleep. Another good tip is to get the baby up for a 'twilight' feed at around 10 or 11pm, trying to wake her as little as possible. With her tummy properly full of milk, and the top-up in the late evening, you might be able to stretch a few more hours' sleep over the night period.

Common Problems and How to Rectify Them

SORE NIPPLES

Sore nipples are one of the most common problems mothers suffer in the early days of breastfeeding and are almost always the result of the baby not latching on correctly. A baby who is not well attached tends to 'nipple' feed rather than 'breast' feed. This makes the nipple rough, red or even bleed (don't think about it, it will make you wince). If you are suffering from sore nipples by all means use books or DVDs to try to correct the latch, but at the same time arrange to go straight to a breast-feeding clinic or call a lactation consultant. Do it immediately, as in do not pass go, do not collect £200. Continuing with a bad latch will just exacerbate the problem, and the pain, so it is essential to solve it immediately and save yourself the tears. If you don't know where to find a clinic you can contact the NCT or the Breastfeeding Network (see pages 268 and 269 for contact details). Alternatively, call your midwife as she will know about local clinics and, in some cases, will be experienced enough to help you herself.

Note that it is not unusual, nor an indication of a problem, if it is just the first few sucks that feel a little tender, or if you are a bit sore the first day or two after solving a latching problem, but anything more than this – anything sharp, or shooting or teeth clamping – counts as an unusually sore nipple and needs a change in latch.

You can use creams to help with sore nipples (see page 208) – these will not solve the problem, but they can help protect the nipple and alleviate some of the discomfort while you work on the latch.

MILK SUPPLY

The amount of milk a baby is getting is often a source of worry for new mothers. In fact, as many as 75 per cent of mothers in the West cite a lack of milk as their reason for giving up breastfeeding. Yet the truth is, this should be the case for only the tiniest proportion of women (as in no more than 1 per cent as in almost nobody!) Not being able to measure exactly the amount of milk that goes in, in ml or ounces, understandably unnerves many women – 'If I don't see it, I don't believe it,' one mother told me – as do all the stories of other women 'who couldn't do it' or 'needed top-ups'. Trust yourself. Whether you choose to breastfeed or not, you are designed for the job. A well-latched baby will get all she needs.

If your baby is genuinely not putting on weight, then it is obviously advisable to contact a midwife or health visitor, but there are also a lot of things you can do to ensure your milk supply is good and accessible to your baby. Remember, if the problem does arise the circle is a vicious one – if your baby is not taking enough milk, your body will reduce its supply, thinking demand has gone down. As with all breastfeeding problems, resolving them early is key.

Once again – and by now you're probably bored of this advice – position is essential. A well-latched-on baby will stimulate the breasts in the right way and activate the let-down reflex. A poorly latched-on baby will send poor signals – by now I am sure you get the drift.

If you feel that your milk supply is dwindling regardless of a good latch, then you might want to start expressing at the end of the day. This will heighten the demand signals and so help to increase supply. Do not be alarmed if you are only getting the tiniest amount of milk when you express. What a lot of women aren't told is that the amount you get from expressing is not the same as a baby would get through its natural suckling. Breast-feeding is hormonally driven. Your baby, and her suckling, activate the necessary hormones for lactation and let-down, a machine does not. And, rest assured, whatever amount of milk you produce when you express, you will be stimulating your body to give you more.

Although the focus is very much on your baby at this time, it is important not to forget to look after yourself. (That is relevant whatever we are talking about – in fact, there is a whole other book in that!) Breastfeeding burns up to 500 calories extra a day. You are likely to be hungry, even ravenous, when you feed, and very thirsty too. Make sure you listen to your body. Diets are not advisable at this stage, even if you are tired of the little pouch at your tummy. Eat healthily and don't miss meals. In fact, it's a good idea to institute a mandatory snack at 4pm to keep your milk supply up for the evening. There is a much bigger gap between lunch and dinner than there is between breakfast and lunch – certainly too long for the usually ravenous breastfeeding mother. So get thoroughly vintage and reinstate the age-old tradition of afternoon tea. Help yourself to a slice of cake or banana bread, or snack on carrots and hummus or a piece of fruit (or both) – and your milk supply will respond.

MASTITIS

Mastitis is either an inflammatory response to poor milk removal, whereby the duct gets blocked, or it is an infection. If you find yourself suffering from mastitis, then it is important to find out what it is caused by so you can treat it appropriately. The inflammatory response doesn't need antibiotics, the infection does. You will know you are suffering from mastitis if you develop an area on one breast that becomes very hot, extremely painful and red. You will also start to get all the symptoms of flu because the milk starts to spill over into the bloodstream and the body treats it like a foreign protein, giving you all the same symptoms as you would have with a virus.

If you suspect mastitis then go to see a breastfeeding specialist. It might be an idea to arm yourself with an antibiotic prescription too, but don't take it until you have tried to establish the cause. The best way to do this is to empty your breast of milk with a pump and take an anti-inflammatory, like ibuprofen (if it is suitable for you). If the symptoms go away and then don't come back, then the cause is inflammation and in all likelihood you need to correct your latch. If the symptoms return, then you probably have an infection in which case it is a good idea to take the antibiotics.

Make sure you continue to breastfeed, as this will drain the breast — there will be nothing wrong with the milk, despite the fact that you feel hideous. You can also express to help clear the duct, directing the machine in such a way that it draws specifically from the area that is blocked. Drink lots of water and take to your bed if you can, getting as much sleep in between feeds as possible. When you have resolved the problem, check your latch again as sometimes mastitis can be the result of an asymmetric latch, in which milk is not being drawn enough in one area. Changing your breastfeeding position – for example, adopting the rugby hold (see page 232) – may also help. Make sure you don't wear tight bras or tight clothes, as this can restrict your milk flow.

FEEDING IN PUBLIC

Although it is often not a problem per se, and certainly shouldn't be, it is surprising the number of women who say they struggle with breastfeeding in public. I had one friend in particular who was very naturally oriented when it came to birth, but never breastfed her babies for more than three weeks or so. She eventually confessed it was because feeding made her housebound, so strong was her discomfort at feeding publicly. Obviously, no one can change the way you feel, but it is important to recognise that breastfeeding is more accepted than you probably think. Boobs that are exposed for feeding are not the same as those exposed as a sexual object, and most people know the difference. Although there is the odd story that hits the headlines of breastfeeding women having been asked to leave somewhere, the truth is most places are breastfeeding friendly. And some places are specifically designated – www.breastfeedingsupport.co.uk lists them by county. Once you are comfortable with breastfeeding, you can throw a piece of muslin or a scarf over your shoulders to enable you to breastfeed discreetly, and it is another reason to get yourself a baby sling – the good ones allow you to feed in them, meaning

Sunday lunch with the in-laws is a breeze! Remember, also, that the more women breastfeed in public, the more accepted it will continue to become in our culture.

AND IF BREASTFEEDING DOESN'T WORK FOR YOU?

If breastfeeding simply doesn't work for you, despite your persistence, then try not to fret. Breastfeeding is an experience fraught with emotion and while some women give it up without a care in the world, others do so with more misgivings. Whatever you do, don't feel guilty – too many mothers do and it is futile. It is still absolutely possible to be a wonderful, loving mum, who gives her baby plenty of love and attention, without breastfeeding. Try to still do as much skin-to-skin contact as you can, as this will give your baby the benefits of bacterial transfer,[34] will help with bonding and will prove really calming to your baby, so bestowing on her a lot of the non-nutritional benefits of breastfeeding.

Remember, working out what is right for you and which paths you and your baby are going to take is all part and parcel of being a mother and, ultimately, there is no single right way to do anything. Don't let anyone make you feel otherwise.

SUMMARY

- The benefits of breastfeeding are very real and well documented so it is worth at least trying to breastfeed in the early days and weeks after the birth. Every day that you manage is of benefit to your baby and to yourself.

- Though breastfeeding is entirely natural, it is still something that we need to learn, especially as feeding in our culture happens very much behind closed doors.

- Start off slowly and be willing to persist as it can take some time to establish.

- If you are struggling in any way, then get help as soon as you can.

- It is essential to get your baby latched on correctly. Get as much help with this as possible at the beginning, as most breastfeeding problems stem from an incorrect latch.

- Persistence usually pays off. Once you have mastered breastfeeding, it is much more convenient than bottle-feeding – no sterilising, no bottles, no running out of formula milk. Plus the milk is free, with you at all times and the perfect temperature.

- Remember that you also benefit from breastfeeding – apart from the health benefits and the convenience, you get a daily dose of oxytocin and prolactin, both of which make mothering easier.

CHAPTER 11

Beyond the Birth
You and Your Baby

'Birth is just the start, parenting's the biggie.'

Lucy Atkins, *Blooming Birth*

'Motherhood has turned me into a funny creature – I have longer arms, and at least two pairs of hands (though this is not enough), lightning reflexes and quite frankly I smell a bit of sick. Every day I worry about things that don't exist, behold – there really are monsters under the bed! Every day I lift my new friend up in the air and smile so hard that I can feel my middles joining in! It's not a bad way to be, is it?'

Letter from a mother I taught, Cat Dartnall

My grandmother used to say 'mothering is the only thing they don't do degrees in'. And if that was true in her day, then it is even more so now. In a time when 'leisure studies' earns you a qualification, motherhood can really feel like the last bastion of muddling through.

It is unbelievably common for women to lament how under-prepared they felt for the first few weeks after birth, even for being a mother in general. All too often we fixate on the birth, preparing with great fervour, only to find that it passes in under a day and then we are faced – suddenly it seems – with a baby that has until this point been little more than an abstract concept.

'The strange thing about being pregnant and being a mother is that although we know that one leads to the other, they are not part of the same psychological thing,' wrote Nigella Lawson in the *Observer*. 'When one friend of mine, shortly after labour, said that she knew that she was pregnant, but why didn't anyone tell her she was going to have a baby, I knew exactly what she meant.'

We assume that motherhood is going to be this thing that comes completely naturally, but the shelves of parenting guides suggest otherwise. Women in other cultures are shocked that we need manuals for something that should be so instinctive, but those same women have probably grown up surrounded by babies and children, very often nurturing them when they are little more than children themselves. In the West, we are more under-prepared than we ever have been throughout history. Often our babies can be the first ones we have ever held, let alone been responsible for. And while mothering is instinctive to a degree, in very large part it is also something that we learn. And for most of us, we only get the chance to learn on the job.

There is a fabulous African proverb that says 'It takes a whole village to raise a child'. Mothers should be just one of many adults who are involved in the nurture of a child. Yet in the West, mothers are very often hundreds of miles from their nearest relatives, and completely devoid of community. No wonder, then, that when the doors close behind the last of the overexcited relatives and dad has gone back to work, a new mother can feel very alone and confused.

Mothering Guides: the Good, the Bad and the Ugly

Enter the manual. Our bookstores are filled with parenting guides of every possible flavour and bent. At one end of the spectrum there are the rigid routines, advocated by the likes of Gina Ford and Tracy Hogg. These proclaim to give women a step-by-step method to get every baby into a routine that ensures they are well fed and sleeping through the night (that Holy Grail of modern times) by the time they are eight weeks old. At the other end of the mothering spectrum are the attachment parenting theories, described by Jean Liedloff, William Sears and Deborah Jackson. These ideas are more baby-led, and involve co-sleeping, feeding on demand and constant carrying of the baby. And in among these two extremes are endless manuals, websites and well-meaning women of every age and opinion, with advice, ideas, old wives' tales and things they did 'in my day'. The problem is all of these imply that there is a single, perfect way to bring up a baby, when in fact there is no such thing. The truth is, there are as many ways to bring up babies as there are children on this planet. What works for one mother and baby might not fit the bill for another. And even the same mother will do things quite differently with different children. While a single workable system would be ideal, the truth is it simply doesn't exist.

Deciding how you are going to mother before you have a baby is very difficult. Whereas you can, to a degree, prepare for birth, being a mother is less about fact and more about feeling. By all means, read the odd book for guidance (see page 267 for recommendations), but try not to take anything as gospel. Everything has a nugget of wisdom in it, and it is perfectly possible to supermarket shop your way through motherhood, using the books as a sort of pick-and-mix affair to suit yourself and your baby (and remember every baby is different, so what works for your first-born might not for the next one or two or three). And be warned, whereas women are often united in pregnancy they can be divided in parenthood. I have heard countless times of women who claim they feel judged by a friend who is doing things by a different book. All too often, advice that is well meaning can seem to be a lecture and there is no doubt that the new mother is a sensitive being. So take advice – be it from books or friends – but be willing to adapt it to suit your own character and that of your baby. If you don't wear a watch and live life rather whimsically it is going to be a struggle to follow the dictates of a rigid routine. Similarly, if you by nature like to plan and organise, you might find a baby easier to absorb into your life if you can gently nudge him or her into a rhythm that you feel you have some control over.

The truth is, when the birth is over and the dust has settled, you will probably feel very differently to how you imagined, and how you mother will probably be unlike what you planned. And rest assured that it will also change over time. You don't suddenly reach a point where you think – aaah, this is it, I have cracked it,

I am now a proper mother. It is an organic process, constantly changing in the same way that we as individuals, and babies in particular, are constantly changing. No matter what 'camp' you fall into, some muddling through will be part of the process, and the best mothers in the world will confess that is exactly what they did, and are probably still doing. A lovely mother in one of my postnatal classes once said to me, quite aptly, 'Everyone needs to become just a little bit of a hippy when they become a mother. You need to be able to just let things be.'

So what comes next is by no means a didactic guide to motherhood. I am not going to tell you what to do or how you should do it, but instead just suggest things you might want to consider when you are thinking about mothering. If nothing else, the exercise is a fruitful way of looking beyond the birth and not fixating entirely on your due date and the 24-hour period that will be your birth and the surrounding time. As everyone always says, birth is just the beginning.

Behind the Scenes

The first thing to consider is what you are actually doing when you are being a mother. While some women completely revel in the simplicity of nurture, others find that they often feel unfulfilled. Many of us are used to ticking boxes and making visible progress. At school we are graded and streamed and congratulated for our achievements. At work we make our way up the rungs of the ladder, or we compare our yearly pay cheque to judge – even just to ourselves – how we are doing. Yet motherhood has no such measures and even the mothers who completely revel in motherhood will have days where they feel overwhelmed and struggle to recognise the value in what they are doing. What's more, once you are over the roller-coaster that is the first few weeks, the charge is often rightly levelled at motherhood that it involves being very busy doing seemingly mundane things. In fact, a friend once described motherhood as being 'everything ad infinitum, ad nauseam'. Whether it is one feed leading into another, the endless hip-swaying to soothe their cries, the non-stop pushing them on a swing or the asking them till you are blue in the face to come to get in the bath, repetition is very often the name of the game. And it is on these days, when you feel like it's been a version of Groundhog Day, that you need to know the intricacies of the endeavour you are undertaking and quite what an extraordinary thing it is that you are doing, even when it doesn't feel like it. Because as boring as it can sometimes look, or as tiring as it might feel, in being a mother you are doing no less than building a little human being, physically, mentally and emotionally – and as anyone who has done it before you will testify to, that is no mean feat.

Babies are born hugely immature. Apparently, to be born with the same level of development as chimpanzees – our nearest animal cousins – we would have to be born at nine months old (youch?!) This means that for a crazy amount of time, human babies are utterly dependent on their mothers. Whereas foals and lambs can walk within seconds, we would survive just a few hours without our mothers. The result is, human mothers have to pull out all the stops simply to keep their babies alive for the nine months that they need to be as developed as a two-day-old monkey! And whether a mother is ultimately 'good' or 'bad', this process alone takes unrivalled energy and commitment. Energy and commitment that is all too often overlooked.

There is a meditation process that Tibetan Buddhists are encouraged to do where they are asked to sit and remember the kindness of their mother. In doing so, they are encouraged to see quite how much nurture it takes to mother, and to then cultivate love and gratitude for their mothers for all their hard work and sacrifice. Then, when they are feeling saturated with love for their mothers, they are encouraged to expand the scope of their thinking, imagining that everyone is or could be their mother and so feel love and compassion for all beings. This has long been a tradition in Tibet and Northern India, and has proven a hugely successful way of altering the mindset of generations of Buddhists. Yet when the monks brought this idea to the West, they were surprised at how many people resisted this particular meditation. 'I can't possibly do this,' people would say, 'I have issues with my mother.' 'My mother was terrible,' others would complain. And yet, as the monks would try to reassure their students, for the vast majority of people, our being here today – our simply being alive – is thanks to an extraordinary effort on the part of our mothers.

Of course, our physical development is just part of the picture. Mothers, in their simple acts of nurture, are in fact doing much more than just keeping their children alive. Developments in science are now allowing us to map the growth of the human brain, providing an insight into aspects of our nature that have, until now, been hidden deep in the recesses of our heads. Love, and our capacity for it – which has always been the preserve of the poet – is now something that can be explained by the scientists. And what they are telling us should free a generation of mothers from the burden of thinking that they toil in vain, because so much is happening to our brains when our mothers nurture us.

A baby is born with about 200 million neurons, most of which are unconnected. It means that we are little balls of potential, full of parts, but those parts need to be put together for us to function properly. These millions of neurons then gradually connect up in response to our early experiences and, in particular, our early relationships. Everything you do with your baby – feeding, holding him close to you, speaking or singing to him, rocking him – in fact, all the things that feel like nothing – create connections in his brain. And it is no exaggeration to say that the better the quality of nurture, the better the connections.

In fact, this is the very reason why nurture and touch are so essential for babies – all too often we understand a baby's need for food and warmth, but consider his need for hugs and touch as secondary. In fact, some misguided child-rearing practitioners have gone as far as to say that we are in danger of spoiling our babies if we hold and hug them too much, yet the truth is quite the opposite. Not only do we help their brain to develop by holding them, but we give them physical strength and good health in the process. In fact, the human need for touch has never been more starkly shown than by a desperately sad study done in Romanian orphanages, where children who were fed and clothed adequately but denied physical contact completely failed to thrive, and many did not even survive.[35]

So be assured you can never love babies too much and that every time you hug them, you are not only soothing them, but helping them become strong, independent people who are more likely to have healthy and happy relationships later in life. It is a huge responsibility, that is for sure, but that you are doing nothing when being a mother could not be further from the truth.

So How Will You Do It?

How will you dedicate yourself to this little human being, and do your very best at making him healthy and happy, without losing your own sanity and sense of self in the process? For that is the key – being a good mother means striking that delicate balance between giving your baby and toddler the intensive nurture that he needs while not completely sacrificing yourself. Of course, we give things up and make compromises in the early years – what job doesn't require sacrifice? But what we need to be thinking of are ways to do it and keep smiling through this short but intense time when we raise young children. As a wonderful early-years teacher by the name of Rita Skit said to me, 'Every family is an ecosystem. The needs of everyone should be in balance.'

GATHER A COMMUNITY

First and foremost, find yourself a community. We used to have them by default but the modern world has changed so that most of us need to artificially construct our community of mothers. But just because we have to find them, doesn't mean they aren't utterly necessary. As soon as you are up and about, hunt around for groups of women who have had babies at around the same time as you and meet up with them on a regular basis. This might not be something you instinctively want to do, but I absolutely promise you, you will not regret it in the long run.

Some women find they have already done antenatal classes and have found kindred spirits in them, while others need to look for postnatal yoga or baby massage classes and for groups who walk together, and then later toddler groups or singing lessons. Thankfully the opportunities are increasing all the time for women to gather with their babies. Midwives and health visitors are a good source of information on what is available in your area.

For many women these groups can, at the beginning, feel a little forced and uncomfortable, especially if you don't fancy yourself as much of a group person or a girls' girl. It can also feel awkward when you feel you have nothing in common with a group of people other than how many times you are being woken up at night and the colour of your baby's poo! But give it time, and these women could well become your lifeline. Women by nature are meant to be in groups. In evolutionary terms, we have always lived like that, with men hunting in packs and women living their day-to-day lives surrounded by other women, sharing the job of cooking, cleaning and nurturing children, while all the time exchanging ideas, seeking support and engaging in idle gossip. The isolated, independent, 10-ball juggling supermum is a thoroughly modern invention. And it is not always that much fun. Having people you can talk to in confidence and seek advice from will make the whole experience of motherhood far less lonely and infinitely less daunting. On a recent trip to Australia, I was at Clareville beach – a magical place on the Northern Beaches in Sydney. One afternoon, a group of women gathered under a tree. There must have been seven or eight of them, and they all had babies that ranged between five and eight months old. While their babies sat and fiddled with grass or made their first tentative attempts to crawl, these women talked to one another constantly. They asked for each other's advice, one of them reassured another about her difficulty with breastfeeding, they laughed together, they spoke about their plans for the weekend. Admittedly none of it was high-brow stuff, yet they all looked happy. Instead of sitting at home, alone, wondering how on earth they were going to while away enough hours to get to bathtime, these women were looking after one another, helping each other to become better mothers.

Obviously many of us don't have access to a gorgeous strip of beach and balmy weather. The local hall or the nearest Starbucks pales in comparison, but the group dynamic, the safety in numbers and the endless wisdom that comes from other women who are – just like you – learning on the job will be no different, no matter where you choose to gather.

BABYWEARING

Secondly, consider babywearing. This is basically using a sling to carry your baby for at least part of the day – though some people get so addicted to the freedom it offers them, and the comfort it gives their baby, that the baby ends up more in it than out; it is for you to decide what works for you. Although it is a practice that is often advocated in the context of very intensive baby rearing, it is in fact something you can do in any context, even if you are using a more obvious routine to help you through the day. Carrying our babies in this way is something Western parents consciously consider doing, yet all over the world babies are carried in this way as a matter of course. In Japan the relationship between mother and baby is considered so close that it is called 'skinship', and among the Ache tribe of Paraguay babies spend a colossal 93 per cent of their day in contact with their mothers. In Bali it is 100 per cent until they are six months old, as there is a belief that if a baby touches the ground before then it will be tainted by the devil. Motivated in part by spiritual belief, and even more by the instinctive sense that close contact with the mother (or any other version of her, be it an auntie, sister, grandmother or friend) will soften the transition from womb to world, babies are held and carried and strapped front or back to their carers. But this practice is also born of necessity. Most women around the world, and especially those in less-developed countries, can't afford the luxury of time that is required to keep a baby entertained but at arm's length. Staying at home while their baby sleeps in a cot in another room is inconceivable. Multi-tasking is essential, and there is no better way to do it than to strap a baby to their back and carry on regardless. And you don't need to be toiling in a field for this to work for you. Wherever you find yourself in the world, and whatever you do, everyone is happy in this scenario. The baby gets exactly what he needs, which is love and nurture and constant rocking and entertainment, while you as a mother get two hands free and an ear that doesn't need to strain for a cry or a whimper. I can honestly say that I am not sure how I would have coped with the demands of three small children had my babies not been in slings.

The concern that it is intense or back-breaking is often voiced by mothers, yet in fact the opposite is true. You will get stronger as your baby gets heavier, so in fact it feels like harder work to carry around a newborn than a four-month-old baby. Your baby will also cry significantly less – in fact, in Jean Liedloff's book *The Continuum Concept* she writes that babies who are carried in slings cry on average for four hours less a day than their Western, arm's-length baby counterparts. Equally, there is less need to explicitly give them attention as they are simply a part of life, happily listening to your heartbeat while being entertained by the world around them and by the constant movement and hubbub of life. Using a sling genuinely gives a mother the ability to have an 'I can take them anywhere' attitude if that's what she chooses. I know babies in slings who have graced music festivals, expensive restaurants, miles of hiking, black tie parties as well as life's more mundane venues like the local park and the aisles of the supermarket. If you feel you'd like to give your baby all the nurture that he might need, but also have to get on and do things, then a sling will be for you.

There are umpteen slings on the market today, in response to what has been a revival in their use. If you are going to buy one, there are a couple of things to look out for. Check, firstly, that you can secure the baby in a number of different positions. This will mean you can use the sling from birth, as the baby can be held across-ways despite lacking strength in the neck. It also means that you can alternate depending on whether the baby is asleep or awake, or if he is quite settled or very windy (a windy baby often likes to be held more upright). In fact, many mothers have told me that the sling was fantastic to use with colicky babies as it soothed them, stretched out their bellies and helped to get their wind up during the difficult 'witching' hour of the early evening. Make sure it is also comfortable for you as the mother – you need a sling that distributes the weight evenly across your back and doesn't pull too much across the shoulders. Finally, make sure you truly can have two hands free and don't need one to secure the baby to you at all times – life one-handed is infinitely more limited!

GIVE YOURSELF A BREAK

Find the time to give yourself a break. In the early days you might not be inclined to, nor feel the need, and that is absolutely fine. It is natural to want to be near your baby almost constantly – nature is no fool. But even in the early days you can allow yourself the luxury of having a long bath and reading a good magazine, and will find that those stolen moments are hugely important. Because being a good mother is so labour and emotion intensive, a little bit of mental space goes a long way to keeping you feeling composed. And then as your baby gets older, follow your own lead and his. If you have family or friends who offer to take him on walks, for an afternoon or even eventually overnight, then when the time feels right, take them up on the offer.

Your Relationships

To say that becoming a mother is life-changing is an understatement by half. I defy anything else to change you as much, and by default to impact so wholly on the relationships you have. Many women say they feel closer to their mother after becoming one, while other people say it brings family rifts to the fore – a previously shy mother might be emboldened by her new role to take a stance on something like never before. Friendships with other mothers can suddenly become more prescient and more meaningful, while you can feel worlds away from other friends whose lives are maybe following different paths. Accepting these changes is part and parcel of the transition to motherhood.

Most acutely felt is probably the change in your relationship with the baby's father, if he is the person you share your life with. In fact, so big and so common is the change that, alongside sleep deprivation, it is the most talked-about subject among new mothers.

Out of instinct and necessity, new mothers tend to focus the vast majority of attention on their baby. It is not something you'll necessarily consciously think about, but the hormones that course through you postnatally – especially when you are breastfeeding, but even when you are not – will ensure your baby is your primary focus. This coupled with sleep deprivation, early mornings and the feeling that you rarely have a moment to yourself means that, for a time, your relationship might take a back seat. You will simply not have the energy and possibly not the inclination to be a wife and lover extraordinaire when you have spent all day attempting to be mother extraordinaire.

It is important to recognise that this shift is natural (the hormones involved in breastfeeding reduce your libido), but also that it won't last forever. A lot of books put pressure on mothers to still have candlelit dinners and focus on their partner, but I think that will in all likelihood make you feel guilty if you're not doing it, and make you think that everyone else is. They're not. Instead of feeling like your relationship has to be a number one priority, maybe think about simply making sure that the wheels keep turning, that you keep things running on a low throttle, so that you haven't lost all sense of each other when you are finally beyond the poo, sick, sleep stage and feel like a mortal woman again. Instead of dinner, have a long lazy breakfast together when you can. Remember babies sleep a lot, and they tend to go back to sleep in the morning, which might give you some time for a flick through the papers and a chat over a croissant. If you have some willing help around, suggest the baby is looked after at lunchtime. You are much more likely to have energy in the earlier half of the day than the latter. A lazy lunch can be just as special as dinner. It is good for you, and very good for your relationship, to eek out just a little time when your mind is not so wholly consumed by your baby.

The first meal out that you and your partner have will probably be spent talking about the little person you've left behind, but knowing he is in safe hands and that you can breathe easy for a couple of hours means that you can focus and give each other what is often some much-needed time. While it's important not to lose yourself in your child, it is equally a natural part of being in a long-term relationship that things ebb and flow. Keep an eye on it all, but don't put yourself under undue pressure. As is always the case, it's the little things that will count – a night curled up on the sofa watching a film together, a text message sent in the day to check how your partner is (and the same goes the other way round, of course), half an hour spent flicking through photos of your endlessly fascinating new baby.

Through all of this early stage, communicating is absolutely key. If something is upsetting you, or one or the other of you is feeling neglected, then it is much more easily solved as and when you are feeling it, rather than nine months down the line when you are going to bed back to back and haven't had a decent conversation in months. If you are feeling snowed under, ask for help. Even the most stoic and bold amongst us need it.

And then there's the whole sex side of things. At around six weeks after birth the health visitor usually comes and talks to you about contraception – I can't tell you how many mothers say this makes them want to laugh out loud. In all likelihood sex will genuinely be the last thing on your mind. It's the one time in your life when contraception is categorically not an issue. But like everything else, gradually your libido will return though don't be at all surprised if it takes some time. If you have had stitches then things will be tender for a while and when you are feeding, your breasts are likely to be no-go zones – even if their new stature seems ever so tempting to your partner! Whatever you do, don't rush into anything. It will all happen in its own time. Think of it as courting all over again – that in itself can be fun!

Banish the Guilt

All too often, mothers – for one reason or another – have episodes of guilt. The mother who works feels bad for leaving her child. The one who doesn't feels guilty that she is not doing more. The mother who leaves her baby to cry feels like she can't tell people she does it, and the mother who is having a bad day and shouts at her lot feels guilty for not being more patient. No matter how much you do, there is very often the feeling that it is not quite enough. And when we get things wrong we are our own worst judges. Perhaps it is one of those crazy parts of the modern mother, that she is expected to do the impossible, so no matter what she does, guilt will be a part of it. It was only the other day that I was having a conversation with a friend through the window of her car. 'How are you?' she asked me. 'Really well,' I responded. 'It's a Thursday and for the first time in 10 years I am having a day off. I am not sure what took me so long to figure out that all I needed was a couple of hours to myself.' My friend just smiled at me knowingly and said, 'It takes about that long to get over the guilt!' It's there, inexplicably, in all of us. And yet it is futile. Give yourself a break, practically and metaphorically. Don't take 10 years to not feel guilty about looking after yourself and giving yourself a bit of time. You'll need it.

When It's All Too Much

The transition to motherhood is undoubtedly enormous and it comes with its fair share of emotional upheaval. The fourth day baby blues are well documented (see page 205) and transient, but it is equally not at all uncommon to have slumps several weeks or months down the line. If it's just a day or two then be gentle on yourself and treat yourself to a long soak in a bubble bath (my cure, it seems, for almost anything) and an early night. If you have a group of mothers you meet with regularly, then think about talking to them too. Be the first person to admit you're struggling and you'll be surprised at how it emboldens others to confess what they are finding difficult too. I can promise you, you aren't alone in having your down days and as that old saying goes, 'A problem shared is a problem halved.'

Sometimes, being on a downer for a few days can slip into something more lingering. In fact, 10 to 15 per cent of mothers develop what is known as postnatal depression (PND). It usually develops within the first four weeks after childbirth, though it can start several months or even a year after the birth. Similar to conventional depression, its symptoms are a low or heavy mood that doesn't want to budge, a feeling of lethargy and difficulty getting interested or excited about anything, coupled with irritability and being teary. In little bursts this can all be considered part and parcel of new motherhood, but if it is persistent it is likely that you are suffering from PND. If you are, or even think you are, then it is really important to get help and it is better to get it quickly. It is not in any sense a sign that you are a bad mother, or that you can't cope while everyone else can. It is much more common than you think, so by no means a taboo any more. Though the exact cause is still unknown, it is thought to be linked to hormonal changes and exacerbated by tiredness – which is another reason to follow the advice of sleeping when your baby sleeps.

Whatever you do, don't bottle it up or try to simply soldier on. There is a huge support network out there to help women with postnatal depression, but you need to go and find it. Before seeing someone it is a good idea to write down how you are feeling – not only is this cathartic in itself, but it can help you gather your thoughts when you speak to someone. Friends, your midwife, your health visitor or your GP can be your first port of call. If you prefer to begin with someone a bit more anonymous, then there are several organisations that are there to help – see page 268. If your low mood is specifically related to the birth, then it might be a good idea to call the Birth Crisis helpline. Whatever happens, try to remember that you will get better and that you are by no means alone.

This Too Will Pass

Finally, remember the old adage 'this too will pass' – in both good times and bad. Those sleepless nights, the endless nappies and the ear-splitting tantrums will all too quickly vanish and before you know it you'll have a hairy, smelly and irate teenager standing before you, who you'll have to hold down to get a hug from. The baby days pass quickly, and the truth is when they are over we very often miss them.

There was an article in the papers many years ago by an Australian journalist, where he described the chaos of Saturdays when there was always a frantic rush in hideous traffic to get his arguing children from one suburb and one sporting activity to another. It was only now, he said, as he sat at his desk in a quiet house, with the children long gone and only the cat for company, that he realised quite how much fun he'd been having.

Relish it all, the good and the bad. Make sure you take time out, in among all the chaos that is bringing up a baby and children, to recognise that you are in the midst of an amazing, overwhelming and extraordinary time. And that you are actually doing it. It can be tough, because our hands are very full, but it is also true to say that with little babies and small children, our hearts are very full too.

SUMMARY

- Mothering is an awesome task that draws on all your resources: physical, emotional and intellectual.
- Remember that even the smallest tasks are part of a much greater whole that is bringing up a baby both physically and emotionally. It is often hard work, but never forget how valuable it is.
- You can never love babies too much, nor spoil them with too many hugs. In fact, science now shows that physical nurture helps a baby's brain to develop.
- Consider babywearing – baby gets the hugs, while you have two hands free.
- Gather a community. The modern mother can be very isolated, yet traditionally children were reared surrounded by a very hands-on community.
- Give yourself a break – mental and physical. You need it, and you deserve it.
- Try to remember that despite the sleep deprivation and the intensity of early motherhood, you will one day look back on this time and marvel at how special it was.

HOW TO COPE WITH LABOUR, BIRTH AND BEYOND

- Believe you can give birth. Trust your instincts and the mantra that your body knows what to do.
- Understand your mind and where it needs to be for birth. Create the best possible conditions for you to switch off that eternally whirring 'front'/intellectual brain.
- Understand your options and be resolute in what you would like. At the same time keep an open mind. Birth won't always go according to plan, but the key is to stay at the centre of your own experience.
- Be as active as you can. Think gravity and a nice, wide, open pelvis.
- Breathe. You cannot hold on and exhale at the same time.
- Hum if you need to – it helps switch off the front brain, which is why monks chant. In fact, make as much noise as you like. There seems to be an inverse relationship between how much noise a woman makes and the discomfort she feels.
- Consider using water. It makes labour shorter, reduces the need for pain relief and enhances the experience of labour.
- Have a doula or another female birth partner. The difference it makes is staggering.
- Be aware of your posture and the positions you adopt during pregnancy. If a baby is in the optimal position at the onset of labour, it makes all the difference.

- Consider intervention carefully. Birth is a delicate balancing act. Upset the balance with care and only out of choice or absolute necessity. Don't be cajoled into or out of anything.
- Do not, under any circumstances, feel you need to justify or apologise for giving birth in whatever way you choose, whether you choose it in advance or in the moment. Guilt is a wasted emotion.
- Let go – physically and mentally. That is what birth is, an act of letting go in every sense. Be willing to let go, even embrace it as liberating. It really is.
- Accept as much help as possible after the birth.
- Give yourself time – to establish breastfeeding, to bond, to get life back on some sort of even keel. You have time, and the baby stage is so short, even if it doesn't feel it at the time. Remember, you are not trying to get anywhere – it's not a marathon.
- Remember that everyone else is muddling through too, and the chances are you are doing a good job of it.

RESOURCES

DESERT ISLAND BIRTH BOOKS

Armstrong, Penny and Feldman, Sheryl, *A Wise Birth* (Pinter & Martin, 2007)

Atkins, Lucy and Guderian, Julia, *Blooming Birth* (Collins, 2005)

Balaskas, Janet, *The New Active Birth Book* (Thorsons, 1991)

Gaskin, Ina May, *Ina May's Guide to Childbirth* (Bantam, 2003)

Gordon, Dr Yehudi, *Birth and Beyond: Pregnancy, Birth, Your Baby and Family, The Definitive Guide* (Vermilion, 2002)

Odent, Michel, *Birth and Breastfeeding: Rediscovering the Needs of Women during Pregnancy and Childbirth* (Clairview Books, 2003)

BOOKS FOR BEYOND THE BIRTH

Gordon, Dr Yehudi, *Birth and Beyond: Pregnancy, Birth, Your Baby and Family, The Definitive Guide* (Vermilion, 2002)

Jackson, Deborah, *Baby Wisdom* (Hodder Mobius, 2002)

Kitzinger, Sheila, *The Year After Childbirth* (Prentice Hall & IBD, 1996)

Stadlen, Naomi, *What Mothers Do; Especially when it looks like nothing* (Piatkus, 2004)

ADDITIONAL INFORMATION

Active Birth Centre – www.activebirthcentre.com
> Fantastic resource, wonderful workshops and good shop.

AIMS (Association for Improvements in Maternity Services) – www.aims.org.uk
> Tel: 0870 7651433
> The place to go if you are struggling to get the birth you want.

Birthchoice – www.birthchoiceuk.com
> Information on hospitals and birthing centres across the UK.

Buddhabellies – www.buddhabellies.co.uk
> Birth blog, comprehensive articles and yoga for pregnancy DVD.

Caesarean Birth and VBAC information – www.caesarean.org.uk

Home Births – www.homebirth.org.uk
> Fantastic resource if you are considering a home birth.

International Caesarean Support Network – www.ican-online.org.uk

NCT (National Childbirth Trust) – www.nctpregnancyandbabycare.com
> Tel: 0870 7703236
> The UK's biggest provider of antenatal care and a comprehensive resource.

YOGA FOR PREGNANCY

Buddhabellies Yoga for Pregnancy DVD by Nicole Croft – www.buddhabellies.co.uk

Freedman, Françoise Barbira, *Yoga for Pregnancy, Birth and Beyond* (Dorling Kindersley, 2004)

IF YOU ARE STRUGGLING POSTNATALLY

(APNI) Association for Postnatal Illness
Tel: 020 7386 0868
Postnatal depression helpline.

Birth Crisis – www.sheilakitzinger.com
Tel: 01865 300266 or 01380 720746 or 020 7485 4725
A helpline set up by Sheila Kitzinger for women who feel traumatised by birth.

FOR DADS

Fathers Direct – www.fathersdirect.com
Tel: 0845 6341328
Good source of information for fathers and fathers-to-be.

FINDING A DOULA

DUK (Doula UK) – www.doula.org.uk
Tel: 0871 4333103

Nurturing Birth – www.nurturingbirth.co.uk

BREASTFEEDING HELPLINE

The Breastfeeding Network Helpline – www.breastfeeding.co.uk
Tel: 0870 900 8787

La Leche League UK helpline
Tel: 020 7242 1278

WATER BIRTH – POOL HIRE

www.waterbabybirthingpoolhire.co.uk/
http://www.thegoodbirth.co.uk/

REFERENCES

1   Okri, Ben, *A Way of Being Free*, Phoenix House, 1997

2   'A Case Report of a pregnant comatose woman', American Journal of Obstetrics and Gynaecology, Sept 2003 189 (3), 877-9

3   *WHO Care in Normal Birth; a practical guide*, 1996

4   Parsons, C. et al. 'Self-reported cognitive change during pregnancy', The Australian Journal of Advanced Nursing. Vol. 9, No.1, September-November 1991

5   *New Scientist*, 'Pregnant Women Get That Shrinking Feeling'. January 11, 1997. Volume 153 Issue 2064

6   *Ina May Gaskin's Guide to Childbirth*, p.170, Bantam Books, 2003

7   Dewees, William P., *Compendious System of Midwifery*, 4th edition Philadelphia, Carey and Lea, 1830

8   *Home Births – The report of the 1994 Confidential Enquiry by the National Birthday Trust Fund* Edited by Geoffrey Chamberlain, Ann Wraight and Patricia Crowley Parthenon Publishing, 1997

9   'Outcome of planned home and planned hospital births in low risk pregnancies: prospective study in midwifery practices in the Netherlands' by T.A. Wiegers, M.J.N.C. Keirse, J. van der Zee, and G.A.H. Berghs, British Medical Journal 23 November 1996; 313: 1309-1313

10   *The Business of Being Born*, 2008, film directed by Ricky Lake and Abby Epstein

11   Engelmann, G.J.: *Labor Among. Primitive Peoples*, 1st ed. St. Louis, Chambers, 1882

12   Enkin M. et al, 'A Guide to Effective Care in Pregnancy and Childbirth' (3rd edition), Oxford (OUP)

      Flynn, A.M, Kelly, J., Hollins, G., and Lynch, P.F. et al, 'Ambulation in Labour', British Medical Journal August 1978 pp.591-593

      Caldeyro-Barcia, R. 'The Influence of Maternal Positions on time of spontaneous rupture of membranes, progress of labour and foetal head compression, Birth and Family. Journal 6:1, 1979, pp.7-15

      Chan, D.C.P. 'Positions in Labour', British Medical Journal 1:12, 1963 pp. 100-102

13 Gestaldo, T.D. 'The Significance of maternal position on pelvic outlet dimensions. Correspondence', Birth 19. 14:230, 1992

14 Gupta, J. (1991) 'The Effect of Squatting on pelvic dimensions'. European Journal of Obstetrics, Gynaecology and Reproductive Biology

15 Andrews, C. and Crzanowski, M. (1990) 'Maternal Position, labour and comfort'. Applied Nursing Research

16 Scott, D.B. and Kerr, M.G. 'Inferior vena caval pressure in late pregnancy', Journal of Obstetrics and Gynaecology, British Commonwealth Vol 70, pp.1044-1963

17 *The Business of Being Born*, 2008, film directed by Abby Epstein

18 Atkins, Lucy and Guderian, Julia, *Blooming Birth*, Collins 2005, p.138

19 Matthews, Gail, 'Written Goal Study'. Dominican University

20 Hodnett, E.D. and Osborn, R.W. 'A randomized trial of the effect of monitrice support during labor: mothers' views two to four weeks postpartum.' Birth 1989a; 16:177-183
Hodnett, E.D. and Osborn, R.W. 'Effects of intrapartum professional support on childbirth outcomes'. Res Nurs Health 1989b; 12:289-297

21 Hodnett, E.D., Gates, S., Hofmeyr, G.J., Sakala, C., 'Continuous Support for Women During Childbirth', Cochrane Review in: The Cochrane Library Issue 3 2007
Kennell, J., Klaus, M., McGrath, S., Robertson, S., Hinkley, C., 'Continuous emotional support during labour in a US hospital. A randomised controlled trial'. Journal of American Medical Association 1991 May 1:265 (H): 2197-201

22 Green, J.M. and Baston, H.A., 'Feeling in control in labour: concepts, correlates and consequences' Birth 30(4), 235-247

23 Thorp, J.A., Hu, D.H., Albin, R.M., McNitt, J., Meyer, B.A., Cohen, G.R. and Yeast, J.D. 'The effect of intrapartum epidural analgesia on nulliparous labor; a randomized, controlled, prospective trial,' American journal of Obstetrics and Gynaecology Oct 1993; 169 (4): 851-8

24 Cluett, E.R., Nikdem, V.C., McCandlish, R.E. and Burns, E.E. 'Immersion in water in pregnancy, labour and birth'. Cochrane Review In the Cochrane Library, Issue 2 2004

25 Gilbert, R.E., Tookey, P.A. 'Perinatal mortality and morbidity among babies delivered in water : Surveillance Study and Postal Survey', British Medical Journal 1999; 319: 483-7

26 Otigbah, C., Dhanjal, M., Harmsworth, G., Chard, T., 'A retrospective

comparison of water births and conventional vaginal deliveries', European Journal of Obstetrics and Gynecology, Volume 91, Issue 1: pp.15-20

27 Eriksson, M., Matlsson, L.A., Ladfors, L. (1997) 'Early or late bath during the first stage of labour: a randomised study of 200 women', Midwifery 13 (3): 146-148

28 *Ina May Gaskin's Guide to Childbirth*, p.143, Bantam books, 2003

29 Odent, M. *Birth and Breastfeeding*, p.34, Clairview Books 2003

30 Eichenbaum-Pikser, Gina and Zasloff, Joanna S., 'Delayed Clamping of Umbilical Cord: A Review With Implications for Practice: Benefits of Delayed Cord Clamping', J. Midwifery Women's Health. 2009;5(4):321–326

31 'Breastfeeding rates in England amongst the lowest in Europe', *Daily Telegraph*, 5th August 2008

32 'Norway Leads Industrial Nations Back to Breastfeeding', Lizette Alvarez, *New York Times,* 21st October 2003

33 Varendi, H. and Porter, R.H. 'Breast odour as the only maternal stimulus elicits crawling towards the odour source'. Acta Paediatrica Vol 90 Issue 4: 372–375, April 2001

34 Babies transfer bacteria and viruses to the mother as they nurse. This results in antibody production in the mother and accumulation of those antibodies in the mother's milk which is then fed back to the baby, and so further protecting it from germs and illness.

35 Zeanah, C.H., Smyke, A.T., Koga, S., Carlson, E. and the BEIP Core Group (2005). 'Attachment in institutionalized and community children in Romania'. Child Development, 76, 1015-1028

WITH THANKS

This book would not exist were it not for the support and wisdom of an enormous number of people. In particular I would like to say thank you to ...

Grainne Fox, my very wonderful agent for her persistence and belief.

To my editors – Miranda West, for commissioning the book and Susanna Abbott, for her guidance and support, as well as all the team at Vermilion for making it happen.

To Janet Balaskas, Liz Murphy and Alice Charlwood for starting me off on the whole birth journey and for their amazing training.

To Annie Francis and Sophie Moorsom, my own midwives, whose gentle ways and exceptional care showed me how birth could really be.

To Naomi Morton for being an inspiration in the world of birth and for agreeing to cast her savvy medical eyes over the manuscript.

To Nikki Jackson, the most fabulous yoga teacher, for keeping me sane and to the Magic Café in Oxford and to Jaffe & Neale in Chipping Norton for being fabulous writing haunts.

And to Mr Millichamp, who all those years back told me I needed to stop walking around the rim and jump into the abyss. This book has – finally – been the jump.

To Jules and Nick for being a true tonic and the best family anyone could ask for.

To Mum, for her infectious *joie de vie* and her endless faith in me, and to Dad, for his focus on family and for having always opened my eyes to the world.

To Jamie, for being a constant source of inspiration and to Immy, for the adventure that has been the last 17 years!

To Danni and Coco, for convincing me that being a doula was a seriously good idea. And to both Sue and Thelma, who are our fairy godmothers, for manning the ship whilst I have tapped away for hours on end.

And last but by no means least, thank you to Skye, Marcus and Cosmo, my very lovely children who give me the best reason to get up every morning. There is not a day that goes by that you don't make me smile in some small way.

Most of all, thank you to Ed, my husband and my best friend, who I simply could not do life without.

Finally, thank you to all the inspirational women that I have guided or cared for; you have taught me more about birth than I could ever teach you.

....

INDEX

Index

....